LICHFIELD FRIAR

PRACTICAL COSMETIC SCIENCE

This book is dedicated to the former and present students of Kingsway College of Further Education, who have helped by experimenting in making new types of cosmetics, blending new colours, and in general giving very helpful suggestions.

Practical Cosmetic Science

Anne Young
Lecturer at Kingsway College of
Further Education

Mills & Boon Limited
London

First published 1972 by Mills & Boon Limited
17–19 Foley Street, London, W1A 1DR.

© 1972 Anne Young

ISBN 0.263.51388.2

All rights reserved. No part of this publication may be reproduced, stored in a retrieval system, or transmitted in any form or by any means, electronic, mechanical, photocopying recording or otherwise, without the prior permission of Mills & Boon Limited

Made and printed in Great Britain by
The Garden City Press Limited
Letchworth, Hertfordshire SG6 1JS

Contents

	Page
Acknowledgements	vii
Preface	viii

Chapter

1 Historical background — 1

2 Materials used in the preparation of cosmetics — 3
1 Waxes and oils — 3
2 Preservatives and antiseptics — 6
3 Antioxidants — 8
4 Colours — 8
5 Perfumes — 10

3 The skin — 17
1 The structure and functions of the skin — 17
2 Skin allergies — 20
3 Care of the skin — 21

4 Cream preparations — 22
1 General preparation; the formation of emulsions — 22
2 Preparation of cosmetic emulsions — 23
3 Cold/cleansing creams — 31
4 Vanishing/foundation creams — 38
5 Nourishing creams and skin foods — 44
6 Astringent lotions and skin tonics — 47
7 Hand cleaning creams — 49
8 Hand creams — 51
9 Sunscreen oils and creams — 55
10 Shaving creams and lotions — 60

5 Other skin cosmetics — 65
1 Bath preparations — 65
2 Deodorants — 69
3 Face and talcum powders — 72
4 Eye cosmetics — 78
5 Lipsticks — 82
6 Beauty masks — 89

6 Hair, nails and teeth — 93
1 Structure and growth of hair — 93

2 Hair diseases	94
3 To keep the hair healthy	94
4 Hair products	95
5 Structure of nails	110
6 Nail care	111
7 Structure of teeth	113
8 Toothpaste	114
7 Cosmetics for the drama group	**117**
1 Greasepaint	117
2 Mixing of colours	119
3 Removal of stage make-up	120
Appendix I Further Reading	125
Appendix II Raw materials	126
Appendix III Perfumes	158
Appendix IV Addresses of suppliers	162
Appendix V Glossary of scientific terms	164
Index of cosmetic formulae	166

Acknowledgements

I am most grateful for the generous assistance given to me by many firms in the cosmetics industries, both with technical help and with the supply of numerous samples for experimental work.

Alginate Industries
Bio Cosmetics Limited
Bush, Boake, Allen, Limited
Butterfield & Company
Rex Campbell & Company
Glovers Chemicals Limited
Honeywell & Stein Limited
International Flavours and Fragrances
Marchon Products Limited
Midland Silicones Limited
Nipa Laboratories
Norda Schimmel International Limited
Proprietory Perfumes Limited
Ronsheim & Moor
Samuelson & Co. Limited
John E. Sturge Limited
Williams of Hounslow
Charles Zimmerman & Company Limited

I wish to thank Mr George Howard, Chief Cosmetic Chemist of Bush, Boake, Allen, for his help, and also Mr Henry Finlay, Head of Science Department of the Beaufoy School, Lollard Street, London, S.E.11, for his encouragement and great help in reading the typescript and for his many helpful suggestions.

I would also like to express my gratitude to the laboratory technicians at the College for their assistance in setting up apparatus.

I am most grateful to Mr Lewis who has made the lipstick mould, without which no stick cosmetics could have been produced, and to Mr J. Christie for the drawing and planning of the mould.

I wish also to express my thanks to Mr Eustace, Head of the Technical Department at the College, for giving me the facilities to experiment in the work of the cosmetics science course, thus enabling this course to develop in the way it has done.

Finally I must express my sincere appreciation for the assistance of Mrs R. Pember who typed several drafts of the manuscript and generally gave great help and encouragement.

Preface

Cosmetics are substances which are intended to cleanse, beautify and generally to impart a sense of well-being. They may be used to hide facial blemishes, to disguise the greying of hair or merely for decorative purposes. Today they are not only used to beautify but also to nourish and condition the skin and hair. Cosmetics such as deodorants and talcum powders can be used to aid personal hygiene. All cosmetic preparations should be innocuous to the skin and stable under all the varying climatic conditions likely to be encountered.

This book has been written primarily for candidates for the C.S.E. examination in cosmetics. However, it could prove useful in the curriculum of an Arts Sixth Form, as a special topic in the Science Sixth, or as a project in the Science Club.

1
Historical background

From the earliest days of civilization, cosmetics have been used by women to make themselves more attractive. The first cosmetics were colourings such as green ore of copper used as an eye shadow, which has been found in burial grounds dating back to 5000 BC, whilst about 1600 BC a mummy of the eighteenth dynasty is reported to have had red dyed hair. There are many references in the Old Testament to women who "painted" their faces. Eastern women used kohl to darken their eyelids and to increase the lustre of the eyes.

In Egypt the art of cosmetics reached its peak in the time of Cleopatra, who used to bathe in asses' milk for the improvement and whitening of the skin, and who used henna for dyeing the finger nails, the palms of the hand and the soles of the feet. Excavations by Egyptologists have also uncovered whole sections revealing beauty shops, with perfumery and cosmetics inside them. In the Bronze Age there was a flourishing and important Cypriot industry of balsam and perfume. Between the ninth and twelfth century AD, the Arabs knew of the distillation of perfumes.

The use of cosmetics in England originated from the Crusades, when the knights returned with prizes from the harems of the East. During the reign of Queen Elizabeth I, toilet preparations played a very important part in social life. These were kept in perfume boxes known as "sweet coffers", which were considered a necessary item of bedroom furniture.

Mary Queen of Scots is stated to have bathed in wine. The civil war brought an end to progress in the further development of toiletries. At the Restoration there was a complete change, and Ladies of the Court used every means of improving their physical appearances.

In France the use of cosmetics followed a parallel course. It was encouraged in the time of Louis XIII, and frowned upon by Louis XIV. With the rise of Napoleon, there was a revival of interest in cosmetics, which were used by Josephine, and the modern cosmetics industry can be traced back to the first decades of the nineteenth century in France. With the development of the great synthetic dyestuffs industry, the cosmetics industry began to develop as it is today.

What is most interesting from the chemical viewpoint is that Lavoisier, the famous chemist, devoted several studies to the development and making of cosmetics. He delivered a paper on these studies to the French Academy of Science, although at that time he was afraid of being considered frivolous, and expressed his very great regret by apologizing to that august body before actually reading the paper. The Academy gave him an excellent hearing.

A passage in a book written by A. Chaplet (and quoted in *Parfum Moderne*, 1929, page 4) on "Un Travail peu connu, de Lavoisier sur le rouge a levres", states that the father of chemistry did not scorn to study the preparation of make-up. He gives at the beginning of his paper, an outline of the history of rouge, and says, "the preparation of a vegetable rouge, far from being a discovery, is, on the contrary, a very ancient custom". Theophrastus speaks of a root known as *rizion*, from which was obtained a dye to rouge the cheeks. Pliny, the naturalist, speaks of a Lydian root similarly employed. Lavoisier then notes in his book that plant rouges had been prepared in the middle ages by Italian perfumers and that French perfumery was indebted to the Florentine practitioners. He also notes the existence of the art in Marie de Medici's Court for the preparation of the plant roots, and quotes some examples, notably that of the preparation of Isa flower rouge.

Lavoisier also confirms that mineral rouges were not used at the end of the eighteenth century, by carrying out analyses of rouges which he bought cheaply from various Parisian shops. "Every time," Lavoisier says, "a rouge is decolorized by spirits of wine, it is a plant rouge. Every time it is decolorized by an alkali it is an animal rouge. If unaffected by both, it is a mineral rouge". Of course, since Lavoisier's time, more accurate methods of analysing have been devised, but it would be well worth trying the experiment on modern rouges.

2
Materials used in the preparation of cosmetics

1 WAXES AND OILS

The word wax is derived from an Anglo Saxon word "Weax". This word was applied to any substances that resembled the plastic material comprising the honeycomb of the bee.
Waxes can be classified as follows:

1   True waxes, which are esters of the higher molecular weight fatty acids and alcohols. An example is beeswax, which is the ester of palmitic acid, $C_{15}H_{31}COOH$, and myricyl alcohol, $C_{30}H_{61}OH$. The formula for beeswax is $C_{13}H_{31}COOC_{30}H_{61}$.

2   Waxes of the ester type, which are nevertheless not true waxes since they contain glycerides, i.e. esters of glycerol and various organic acids. Glycerol is an alcohol of comparatively low molecular weight when compared with myricyl alcohol. Glycerides are either oils or fats and the latter have a wax-like appearance. Japan wax is an example of this kind of wax.

3   Mineral or hydrocarbon waxes.

4   Synthetic waxes.

5   Waxy substances such as (a) hydrogenated oils (e.g. hydrogenated castor oil) and (b) higher alcohols such as cetyl alcohol, $C_{16}C_{33}OH$, known as lanette wax.

Waxes may be obtained from animal, vegetable and mineral sources. Several are used in the making of cosmetics.

Animal waxes

Beeswax: Ordinary beeswax comes from the honey bee. There are several varieties, the oldest one being the Indian bee. Other important varieties are found in the West Indies, Australia and Italy. Pure wax from the honeycomb is known as virgin wax. The wax is first drained from the combs, separated from the honey and melted over water and poured into moulds. In this form it is supplied to the manufacturers for processing. Two grades are produced—the yellow, which is the natural colour, and the white wax, which is bleached by exposure to the sun or by using chemical bleaching agents such as potassium dichromate and sulphuric acid. The white grade is an important constituent of many creams, lipsticks and eye make up. It contains 11–13% hydrocarbons and about 13% free fatty acids.

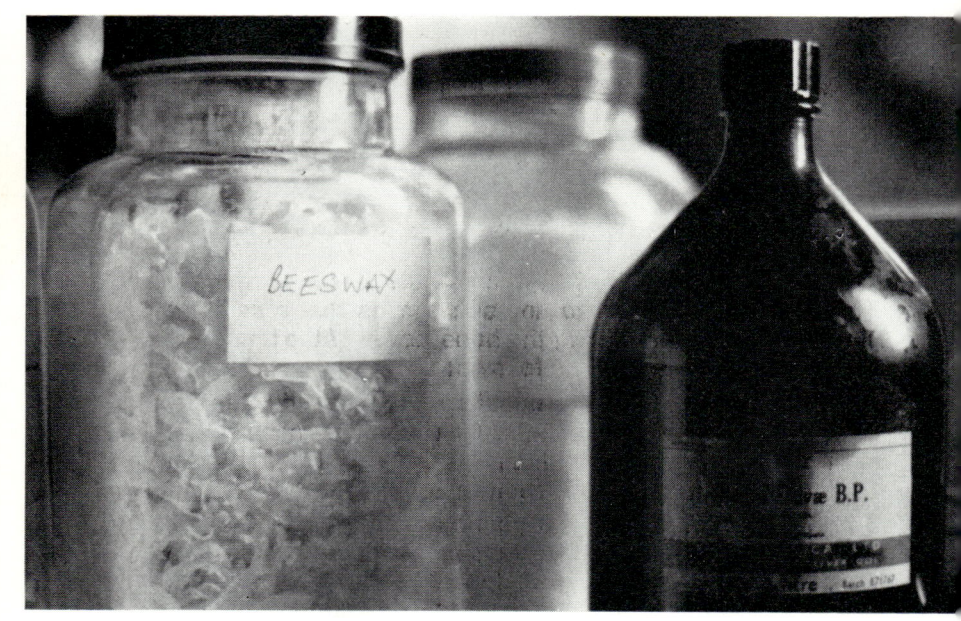

Fig. 1   Raw materials: beeswax.

Lanolin: This is a very good emulsifier and is used in cosmetics. It is a fatty material found in sheeps wool. The wool is treated with a dilute solution of soap and washed, and then treated with dilute sulphuric acid which helps to decompose it. This gives a pure lanolin which is used in the production of cosmetics as an emollient. Lanolin is a complex mixture of water and wax esters. It has many derivatives.

Walrat (Spermaceti): The chief constituents of spermaceti are cetyl palmitate and cetyl myristate. The sperm oil is obtained from the head of the sperm whale and the dogling oil from the bottlenose whale.

The oil is chilled and allowed to stand, the spermaceti separates out and can be removed by filtration. It is a white translucent mass and is odourless and tasteless. It is insoluble in water.

Spermaceti is used in cold creams to improve their gloss and to stabilize the emulsions.

Vegetable waxes

Carnauba: This comes from the leaves of the carnauba palm, found in Brazil, which grows to a height of about 35 feet. The wax exudes from the leaves and forms a greenish grey substance on both sides of the leaves, and is removed by shaking the tree. The leaves are cut from the trees about early September and brought to a forest for cleaning and drying. They are turned over several times a day for about one week. The wax is then collected and melted down, and forms a dark grey mass. If less dirt is left in, the wax is a pale yellow colour. This wax is classified as flower type and is the purest form with over 99.32% of wax. The melting point is 84°C. Carnauba is used in lipsticks to give hardness and solidity to the consistency.

Candillila: This is found as a coating on stems of certain Mexican plants which grow wild. The plants are collected, cut into small pieces and boiled in water to which has been added some sulphuric acid. The wax then comes to the surface and is skimmed off. It is then placed in a tank of hot water for more washing and this process is repeated several times. The wax is then poured into moulds. Candillila is hard and brittle and has a medium brown colour, but can be bleached white. It is used with carnauba to increase the melting point of stick cosmetics in particular.

Wax-like fats

Japan wax: This wax is found in the berries of a small sumae tree which is grown in the East. It is obtained from the berries by drying and hot pressing. The wax is treated with steam and extracted by a suitable solvent. It is a pale, lightly tinted tallow or grease. The melting point varies between 45–125°C.

Mineral or hydrocarbon waxes

Paraffin wax: This consists of purified solid hydrocarbons obtained from petroleum. The finished wax is sold either in the form of soft paraffin wax, petroleum jelly (yellow or white), or in blocks. The wax has a melting point of 50–57°C.

Ozokerite: This is a natural bituminous product. It occurs in the form of a dark brown, yellow or white amorphous wax found in many parts of the world, near petroleum springs. It may be purified by boiling with water. The melting point is in the range 60–72°C.

Cetyl alcohol: This has waxy properties. It is found in the free state as well as in the ester form in spermaceti. It has a melting point of 47–49°C and is soluble in alcohol.

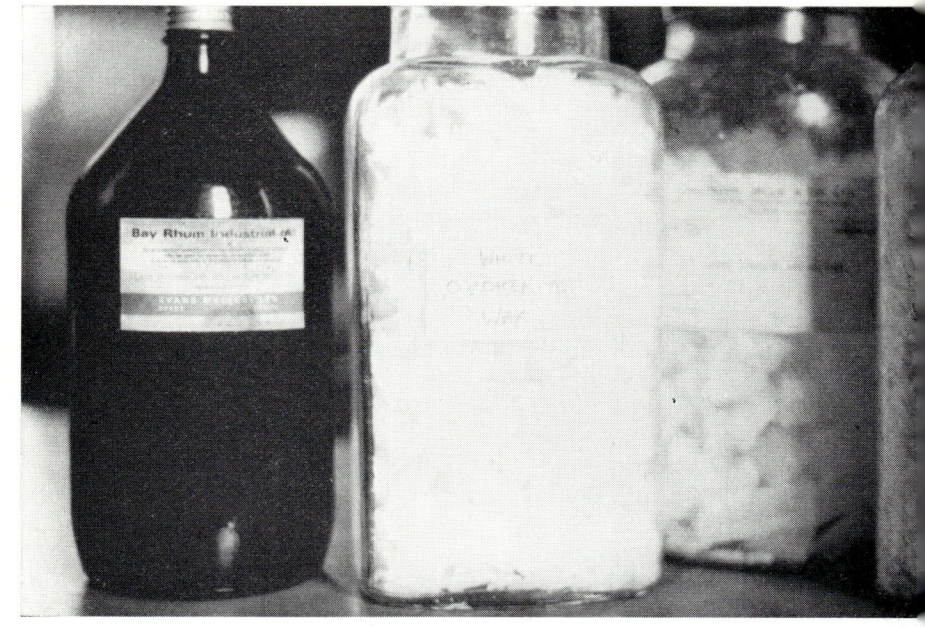

Fig. 2 Raw materials: ozokerite and bay rum.

Properties and functions of waxes for cosmetic purposes

1 They form a water-repellent film.
2 They are oil soluble and, therefore, improve the emolliency of the film left on the skin.
3 They can act as emulsifying agents or auxiliary emulsifiers.
4 They are thickening agents and improve the texture and smoothness of emulsions.
5 They give good gloss and moulding properties for lipsticks.

2 PRESERVATIVES AND ANTISEPTICS

Cosmetic preparations which contain oils and fats must be protected against the growth of moulds and from becoming rancid (rancidity shows itself in bad odours and discoloration of the preparations). To prevent this taking place, preservatives and antiseptics are used. A *preservative* is a substance which prevents the decomposition of the preparation by discouraging the growth of bacteria and fungus. In this way it preserves the colour and odour. An *antiseptic* is a substance which will prevent the growth of bacteria by killing the organism. It is however, used only in preparations which are applied to living tissue. Moulds grow where there is access to the air, as they are aerobic. Therefore, a piece of waxed paper or foil should be placed on the surface and the lid of the jar should be well screwed on.

The materials used for preserving the cosmetic preparations from spoilage by micro-organisms are substances whose main function is to prevent the multiplication of bacteria and fungi throughout the period of use of the creams. The most common mould is penicillin. Separation of the emulsions, liquefaction of the gels and the appearance of small lumps in the cream indicate bacterial infection of the product.

Suitable preservatives for emulsions are the Nipa esters such as Nipagin M, Niposol M and Nipabutyl. These are non-toxic. Solutions of Nipagin M, Niposol M and Nipabutyl can be made in water, alcohol, glycerine and essential oils. Heat the water, add the Nipa and stir constantly until the oily globules, first formed, are dispersed.

SOLUTIONS

In water

2.5 g of Nipagin M
or 0.7 g of Nipagin M
or 0.3 g of Niposol M

are added to 1 kg of water. These can then be used hot or cold.

In alcohol

Four parts of alcohol are needed to dissolve one part of Nipa ester at 25°C.

In fats and glycerine

Warm the Nipas and fats to 70°–80°C.

Other preservatives that can be used are Nipastat, a white crystalline powder which is very stable in aqueous solution, and Nipasef which has the following special applications:

Almond milk	0.18%
Bubble bath preparations	0.14%
Cosmetic solutions	0.14%
Shampoos (cream)	0.20–0.25%

3 ANTIOXIDANTS

These are used to prevent the oxidation of certain materials in cosmetic preparations, for example the common fats such as castor oil, corn oil, mineral oil, etc.

The properties of the antioxidant should be,

1 that it has no odour, as this would interfere with the perfume added to the preparation,
2 that the cosmetic preparation should not deteriorate if kept for some time,
3 that it should not be toxic, and
4 that it should be colourless.

A suitable antioxidant is Progallin. This can be used suitably in minute quantities in preparations which contain almond oil, araches oil, castor oil, olive oil, sesame oil, etc.

The antioxidant is dissolved in the oil phase by warming up to $60°-70°C$.

4 COLOURS

Colours that can be used in cosmetic formulations can be divided into two classes according to whether they are soluble or insoluble. This is most important in the finished cosmetic.

Soluble colours

These can be water-soluble, alcohol-soluble or oil-soluble colours. The three groups of soluble colours are, for the most part, synthetic organic dyestuffs. A dye can be defined as a colorant which imparts its colour only in solution, the solvent being water, alcohol or oil. The soluble organic dyes can be sub-divided into a number of other groups, according to their properties. The most important for cosmetic colouring are:

1 Acid dyes: These are used for dyeing silks, cottons and other materials They are the largest group of dyes and are also used for cosmetics, foodstuffs and varnishes. The characteristic feature of acid dyes is the presence of an azo-group in the molecular structure. These dyes may be blue, green, red, violet, or yellow.

2 Solvent dyes: These are soluble in either alcohol or water. Examples are DC red, green red (No. 17), violet, yellow.

3 Xanthene dyes: These are used in lipstick colouring. Examples are DC orange, red and yellow.

* *

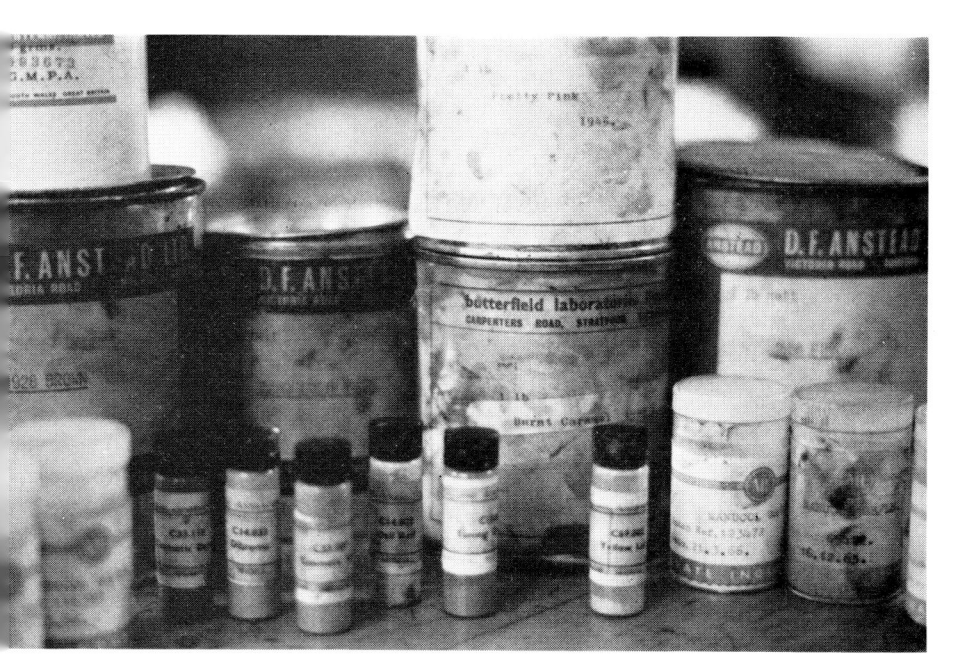

Fig. 3 Raw materials: colours.

Insoluble colours

These can be divided into organic compounds such as the lake dyes and pigments, and the inorganic dyes such as the oxides of certain metals, e.g. ultramarines, greens, blacks, and the metallic colours.

1 Lakes: A lake is a coloured precipitate produced by adsorbing a dye (mordant) on the surface of a metallic oxide or hydroxide. For precipitation of acid dyestuffs, barium chloride is used. Coal-tar dyes used in lakes can either be acidic or basic.

2 Natural iron oxides: Yellow ochre, found in France, Italy, Spain, Cornwall. The iron oxide is found in the yellow hydrated form.

3 Raw and burnt sienna: These are mined with ochres and have a higher content of iron(III) oxide (Fe_2O_3) and a lower content of alumina. Siennas have a manganese oxide content of $1-1\frac{1}{2}\%$.

4 Natural red oxides of iron: These are found in France, Spain, U.S.A. and South Africa. English red oxides have a brownish colour. Natural red oxides contain about 75–90% Fe_2O_3.

5   **Raw and burnt ambers:** These are mined in Cyprus, Italy and the U.S.A. They have a greenish colour and contain 8–16% manganese(IV) oxide.

Organic colours

Blacks—carbon blacks (lampblack), vegetable blacks and bone-blacks.

Aluminium powders

These are used in eye shadows and are made by rolling and beating aluminium into sheets.

Bronze powders

These are copper and alloys of copper reduced to a powder.

All colours must be carefully chosen as the ingredients used in a formula may have an effect on the particular colour. For use in the preparations in this book, colours may be obtained from the manufacturers (see Appendix II). Leaflets can also be obtained, indicating for which preparations these colours are suitable.

5 PERFUMES

The work of the perfumer calls for a great deal of skill and patience. It is a very old profession. The perfumer has to know all about the essential oils, the gums and resins, etc. Perfumes are regarded as a luxury and their use dates back to antiquity. The Greeks and Romans perfumed their wines with violets and roses. The Romans later on boasted of a long list of aromatic medicines. However, it is to the Moslem scientists that we owe the introduction of the systematic distillation of perfumes in the middle ages. Spices which were collected by caravans of Asia from all over Europe were distributed and shipped by the fleets of the Venetian merchants.

Early sources of valuable aromas were provided by resinous gums which were obtained from certain shrubs and trees when the barks of the trees were cut. These gums, when burned, gave off a very strong perfume (incense). Other aromatic materials of antiquity were essences from flowers and fruit juices. These odours consisted of natural vaporous substances which are now called essential oils, i.e. light spirits which evaporate easily and affect the sense of smell. Essential oils are found all over the world. Some flowers and herbs have been gathered in great quantities, but have yielded only a small amount of oil.

Odour of perfume

A perfume is a blend of odorous materials which give an impression of smell. The smell cannot be detected until the vapour is brought into contact with the sensitive lining of the inner nose. This is the olfactory membrane, which is covered by a thin layer of fluid, and when the smell-bearing vapour is dissolved by the fluid in the nose (which occurs immediately), the nerve ending in the olfactory membrane registers the nature and existence of the smell. The nostrils do not register any smell whatsoever; they are merely filtering tubes.

Sources of perfume

The basic materials used by the perfumer are the essential oils. However, there are other materials the perfumer needs:

1. Essential oils in a volatile form derived directly from plants.
2. Gums and resins derived from the bark of trees.
3. Animal scent-yielding products.
4. Indirect products—synthetic and natural.

1 Essential oils: These are very volatile (i.e. they vaporize readily) vegetable oils which are obtained from flowers, fruit, leaves, shrubs and roots. An essential oil is usually obtained from a particular part of a plant, for example:

> Flowers — rose, lavender, orange blossom.
> Seeds   — caraway, almond.
> Leaves — bay, thyme, patchoull.
> Wood   — sandalwood, cedar, aloe.
> Bark   — cinnamon, cascarilla.
> Fruits   — lemon (citron), nutmeg.

These oils come from all over the world—sandalwood (which is very expensive) and lemon grass from India; rosewood from South America; roses from Bulgaria, North Africa and France (when distilled, known as attar of roses); peppermint from the U.S.A.; lavender from England and France and rosemary from Spain, to name a few. The soil and the climate are very important in growing the essential oil-giving plant.

2 Gums and resins: These do not vaporize, but they do contain a certain amount of volatile oil which can be dissolved out of them.

3 Animal products: These are musk, civet, ambergus and castor. *Ambergus* is formed in the intestines of the sperm whale. *Musk* comes from a small gland situated near the sex organs of the male musk deer. *Civet* is obtained from the civet cat. *Castor* is obtained from a secretion of the beaver.

4 Synthetic chemicals: As the demand for more perfumes continues, synthetic materials are being used more and more in place of natural substances. The synthetics are organic chemicals, and are used in all types of perfumes. They consist of the aromatic alcohols and the fatty alcohols, which usually have soft odours, and certain esters and aldehydes. Here are some examples:

1 *Phenyl ethyl alcohol,* which is one of the basic constituents of rose perfumes.

2 *Cinnamyl alcohol*, which is a fixative* and is used in lilac perfumes.

3 *Terpineol,* which occurs in pine oils, but is manufactured from turpentine, an essential oil. It has a woody lilac smell.

4 *Amyl cinnamic aldehyde*, which has a floral odour and is one of the basic constituents for jasmine perfumes.

5 *Esters*, which can be recognized by their characteristic fruity odour. Examples are methyl phenyl carbinyl acetate which is used in jasmine and gardenia perfumes, and benzyl acetate which is used in floral perfumes.

Methods of extraction of perfumes

There are five methods of extraction:

1 Distillation
2 Extraction by solvent
3 Expression
4 Enfleurage
5 Maceration

1 Distillation: This is the oldest method and is applied to plants whose odour will not be destroyed by steam. The materials are either placed in a still filled with water, or steam is passed directly into them from a boiler. The boiling water or steam penetrates the plants, breaks down the cell walls and reaches the tiny droplets of essential oil secreted in the vegetable matter, causing them to vaporize. These two vapours, that is the water vapour and the essential oil vapour, are then passed into a condensing chamber whose sides are kept cool by a current of cold water. Inside the chamber, the mixed

---

* The fixative, in perfumes, causes the ingredients to evaporate at the same rate and so ensures that the odour of the perfume remains constant.

vapours liquefy and the mixture flows into a separating flask where the water and oil automatically separate.

Fractional distillation could also be used. In this case the essential oil is heated and the temperature is raised by stages, when a different chemical component of the essential oil will vaporize at different temperatures. If each of the vapours is captured individually and then condensed to a liquid, it is found that each liquid is a fraction of the mixture which formed the original essential oil.

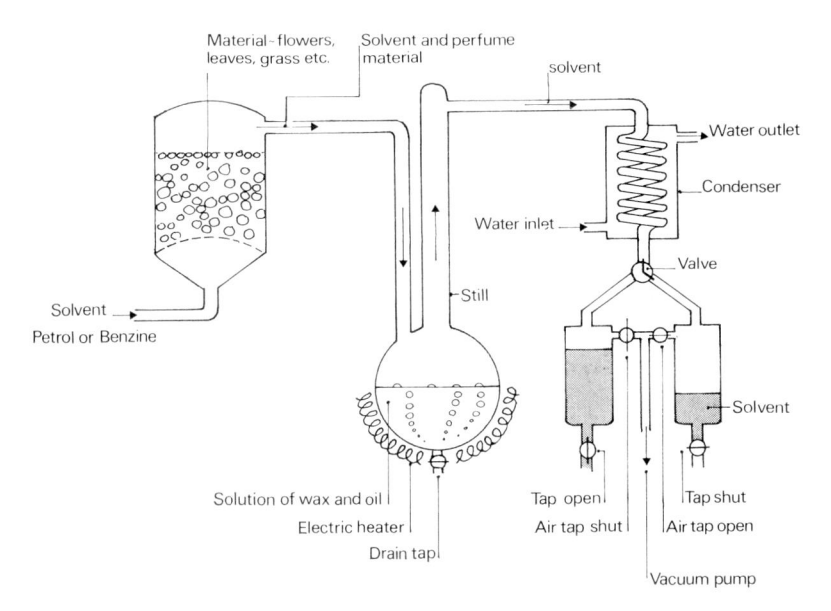

Fig. 4 Diagram showing the process of solvent extraction of perfume. The material is placed in the left-hand container and a spirit solvent is added. The solvent together with a mixture of wax and essential oil runs into the lower half of the still. Gentle heat from an electric heater is applied and the solvent is distilled off, leaving behind in the still a mixture, or "concrete", of wax and oil which is drained off later. The solvent is condensed through the cooling tube and collected in two receivers, one of which is closed while the other is being emptied.

2   Solvent extraction (see Fig. 4): In this method, fresh plant material is placed in a container which is sealed down and is flooded with the liquid solvent (such as ether or petroleum). This evaporates at a low temperature. The solvent then penetrates the plant tissue and dissolves out the essence together with some colouring matter and waxes. The solution is then pumped out and the solvent is removed by evaporation under reduced pressure. The substance left behind consists of waxes mixed with the floral essences. The wax is separated, leaving a liquid which is concentrated essential oil.

3   **Expression:** This is a very simple method. The skins of citrus fruits (such as lemons, oranges and bergamots) are pressed cold to obtain the essential oils.

4   **Enfleurage:** This method uses cold fat, as fat will absorb essential oils. A thin layer of fat is spread on a sheet of glass which is held in a wooden frame. Freshly picked flowers are spread over the fat and left for twenty hours. After this time the flowers have given up their oil to the fat and begin to wither. The frame is then turned over and the flowers fall off. The remainder of the flowers are picked off by means of forceps. A further layer of freshly picked flowers is strewn on the fat and this process is repeated for about seventeen days, depending on the type of flower. In due course the fat absorbs the flower perfume and it is then known as pomade. This is washed in alcohol until all the perfume is transferred to the alcohol, which is then evaporated under vacuum pressure in a cold still, leaving the concentrated flower oil.

5   **Maceration:** After picking, most flowers do not generate essential oils unless they are plunged into hot fat. The hot fat penetrates the cells and absorbs the essential oils in about one hour. The used flowers are removed and further flowers are immersed in the fat. This is repeated about eight to fourteen times. The essential oils are recovered in the manner described in the previous paragraph.

A perfume is composed of various constituents which are called notes. A scale of 1–100 is used, based on an assessment of the volatility of the substances. This is done by noting the time taken for a substance to evaporate completely from a slip of paper.

The *Top Notes* are the most volatile, ranging from 1 to 14, and are first noticed when the perfume is smelled—e.g. citrus oils. The *Middle Notes* range from 15 to 60 and are the blending agents which give body and character to the perfume—e.g. Terpenes, which are oxygenated derivatives of alcohols and their esters. The *Base Notes* are the least volatile components, ranging from 60 to 100, and contain musk or vanillin for balance.

A certain period of ageing is required before an alcoholic perfume can be bottled and ready for use. When the perfume is maturing it acquires a balanced odour. Any fats or wax particles originating from natural extracts are precipitated. This ageing takes two months. Maturation of the perfume is due to a chemical reaction between the components, together with the maturation of the spirits.

Alcoholic perfumes can only mature in glass bottles. Air and light must be excluded. They must be cooled for at least twenty-four hours in a refrigerator before they can be filtered, and should be kept as cold as possible before filtering.

Filtration can be carried out with filter paper and a glass funnel. Synthetic dyes should be added before filtration.

Some formulae are given here and the student may like to try making these. However, these are not suitable for use in the preparations described in later chapters, and it is advisable to obtain perfumes from the manufacturers (see Appendices II and III). Leaflets are also available indicating the preparations for which each perfume is suitable.

Alcohols used in perfumes

A highly rectified alcohol of 95–96% strength should be used with a denaturant of 5% wood-naphtha. Masking the odour of the alcohol is achieved by adding a masking agent (e.g. diethyl phthalate) and then allowing the perfume to mature. Alcohols made from molasses or rice are most frequently used in perfume preparation.

As much distilled water may be added to alcoholic preparations as is compatible with the solubility of the sweet smelling oils used.

Formulae *Grammes*

1 *Toilet Water*
   Toilet spirit   24.00
   Lavender (infused)   0.08
   Oil of bergamot   1.20
   Oil of lavender   2.00
   Infusion of musk pods   2.00
   Infusion of civet   2.00

Method : Mix together. Filter if necessary

2 *Toilet Water (No Alcohol)*
   Distilled water   50.000

Oil of lavender	0.500
Oil of bergamot	0.015
Oil of lemon	0.015
Oil of cassia	0.015

Method: Dissolve the oils in the water and filter.

3. *Toilet Water (Alcohol)*

Toilet spirit	171.50
Oil of lavender	3.00
Oil of bergamot	0.40
Oil of lemon	0.40
Oil of cloves	0.25
Oil of sweet orange	0.10
Distilled water	21.50

Method: Dissolve the oils in the alcohol. Add the water, stir and filter.

4. *Rose Perfume*

Geraniol	30.0
Rhodinol	20.0
Citronellol	10.0
Phenyl ethyl alcohol	40.0

Method: Weigh each oil very carefully. Mix the oils in a glass beaker thoroughly in order to obtain a uniform mixture. If heat is required, this must be done very carefully over a water bath.

Note: If other rose odours are required, add musk ketone or xylol (up to 4% of the total volume) or phenyl ethyl acetate (1–2% of the total volume). The addition of a very small amount of phenyl ethyl alcohol will improve the odour.

3
The skin

1 THE STRUCTURE AND FUNCTIONS OF THE SKIN

The skin is the largest organ of the body and it covers a very large area. It varies in thickness in different parts of the body. It is thickest on the soles of the feet and the palms of the hands. It is a resistant elastic tissue. It becomes thinner and more wrinkled in old age and assumes a yellowish or greyish shade. The cells of the skin are thinnest on the face; this is important for the using of cosmetics which must be able to penetrate the skin.

The skin is composed of two layers—the *epidermis* and the *dermis*, which is the true skin. (See Fig. 5)

The *epidermis* is composed of an outer layer of dead, flat cells of the stratified corneum. These cells have no nuclei and are constantly being shed. They contain a special fatty material which makes the cells waterproof. The lowest layer of the epidermis (the Malpighian layer) is always dividing in a plane parallel to the surface of the skin and thus new layers of cells are always appearing to replace those rubbed off the outside.

The colour of the skin varies with race, climate, season and manner of living. In addition to melanin, which is the most important of the skin pigments, other substances contribute to the colour of the skin. These are carotene, which is a yellowish pigment found mainly in the dermis, melanoid, which is similar to melanin, blood pigments such as haemoglobin, and the subcutaneous fats.

The relative amount of melanin accounts for the difference in the skin colour. A black or very dark brown skin has a larger quantity of melanin in the epidermis, whilst the absence of melanin in fair skin allows the blood pigments to be seen.

The *dermis* is the true skin and consists of fibrous protein, collagen, which is a very tough elastic tissue. The true skin is richly supplied with blood vessels and nerves; it contains the sweat glands, sebaceous glands and the hair follicles. The layer of cells in direct contact with the epidermis are pigment cells. These are also found in the hair follicles around the papilla. It is in these cells that the pigment melanin is formed by a process of oxidation.

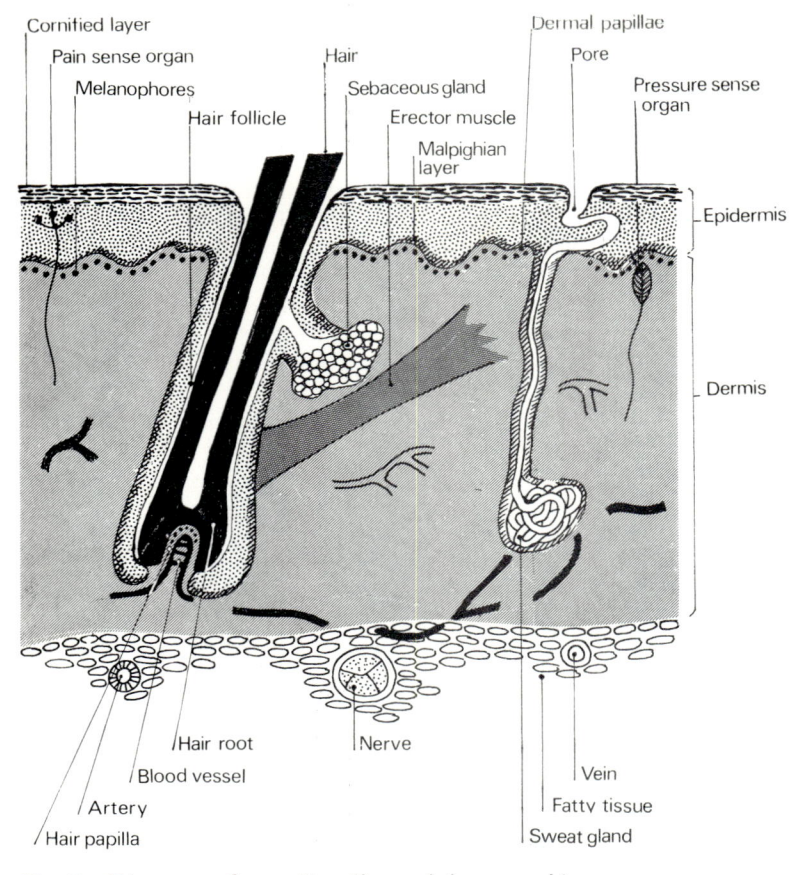

Fig. 5   Diagram of a section through human skin.

The *sebaceous glands* are very small sac-like structures which are open into the hair follicle. The glands are found all over the body, except on the palms of the hands and the soles of the feet, and between the fingers and toes. They are most numerous on the face and the scalp and they secrete an oily substance, sebum, which helps to lubricate the skin and the hair shaft. Sebum consists of various fatty acids, waxes and hydrocarbons (which are compounds composed of hydrogen and carbon).

The *sweat glands*, which are found all over the body, are very coiled. There are two types—the *ecrine* glands which secrete a clear watery liquid which helps to maintain the body temperature, and the *apocrine* glands which secrete a fluid which is composed of nitrogenous products and fats. When it dries on the skin, it leaves a solid residue. If this becomes contaminated by bacteria, it decomposes and leaves a very unpleasant odour. The condition of the skin is due to the state of the surface cells, the activity of the secreting glands and the state of the fatty tissue.

The *pH of the skin* (i.e. the hydrogen ion concentration) varies with the individual and it varies in different parts of the body, according to the time of day. It can also be affected by the type of food eaten during a meal. The skin is less acid in the areas where there is no access to the air. The secretions from the sebaceous glands form the principal element of the acid mantle on the epidermis which has a pH of between 5 and 6. The pH of the skin is frequently higher on the wrist and the forearm than elsewhere.

Some chemicals contained in the skin are certain amino acids such as glycine and valine, fats, mineral salts and a great deal of water.

The functions of the skin. The epidermis prevents bacteria entering the true skin. The outer layer also protects against physical injury, and because of its continual growth and repair, the skin is kept in good condition. The skin is also waterproof and it regulates the body temperature. The skin contains a large number of chemical compounds, e.g. cholesterol and ergosterol which, by the action of ultra violet rays, manufacture vitamin D.

The beauty of the skin is conditioned by the state of the keratinized surface cells, the activity of the secretory gland and the state of the fatty tissue. The surface of a neglected skin is covered with small white scales with raised edges.

Ageing of the skin is due to changes which take place in the dermis. There is a loss of elasticity in the collagen fibres which is due to loss of moisture. There is also an increase of the pigmentation of the skin; brown spots appear and this is due to changes in the oestrogen secretion of the ovary. Too much sunlight can also contribute to the skin becoming older looking. The use of emollient creams and moisturizing creams keeps the outer layer of the skin soft and supple.

Freckles: These are localized collections of pigment which form part of the protective mechanism of the skin. They are found mostly in blond and red headed people and certain people with very light brunette complexions. The melanin is not evenly distributed through the skin and occurs in clumps. Freckles can be inherited.

Moles, too, are usually inherited and are present in the skin in small numbers. A mole is a collection of naevus cells within the dermis. The precise nature of the cells is not known, but they are related to the epidermal melanocytes.

Warts are caused by a virus, which can be passed from one person to another.

The different types of skin: The skin can be classified into four major types—'normal' skin, oily or greasy skin, dry skin (dehydrated) and very dry skin. *'Normal' skin* is firm, smooth, and has a healthy colour and tone. The pores of the skin around the nose and chin are slightly enlarged and there is a tendency to find thin lines around the eyes, mouth and the throat. *Oily or greasy skin* is the type in which the fatty secretions from the sebaceous gland are most abundant around the forehead, nose and chin areas. The pores of the skin are enlarged and there is sometimes a tendency for the sides of the nose to flake. This type of skin has a tendency to blackheads, blemishes and pimples. This type of skin is mostly of an alkaline nature.

Dry skin or dehydrated skin is fine textured and has the appearance of dry parchment with a tendency towards scurvy. It wrinkles easily, showing lines around the eyes, throat and mouth. There is also a shortage of acid. The process of assimilation in the body of the food that is consumed contributes to this type of skin. *Very dry skin* has a parched, thirsty look and is of a very fine texture, with sometimes broken veins. It is sensitive to cold. This type of skin shows deep wrinkles and a tendency to loss of firmness in the facial contours.

2 SKIN ALLERGIES

An allergy is a reaction between an antibody (protein substance) and antigens. Certain factors can contribute to skin allergies, viz. the use of synthetic perfumes instead of natural perfumes, and the widening range of chemical compounds used in making various preparations. Some of these compounds, known as sensitizers, can cause skin irritation which affects only certain individuals.

The most common disease of the skin is dermatitis. If certain preparations are used, the skin becomes red and begins to swell. There is a tendency for the skin to crack and there is a slight irritation. The papillae (which consist of a mass of dermal tissue, containing blood vessels and nerves, covered with epidermal cells) begin to rise.

One of the more common forms of cosmetic sensitivity is lipstick dermatitis. This is due to the eosin, which is the staining ingredient in the lipstick. In some people the lips become inflamed after they have been exposed to the sun—the eosin has sensitized the lips to the sun's rays, and this is known as photo-sensitization. To overcome this, the eosin can be omitted from a formula and a barrier cream can be used on the lips before lipstick is put on. Some people are sensitive to perfumes, whether essential oils or the synthetic perfumes. Perfumes should not be used in such cases.

Acne is connected with excessive activity of the sebaceous gland and the secretion of a great deal of sebum which makes the skin very greasy. Therefore, cosmetics which contain a lot of fat should be avoided, particularly in the cleansing of the skin. A lotion which contains a mild antiseptic agent, e.g. cetrimide, is more suitable for cleansing very greasy skin.

3 CARE OF THE SKIN

In order to ensure that the skin is kept in good condition, the following practices should be adopted:

1   Cleansing.
2   Freshening or toning.
3   Moisturizing.

To clean the skin it is better to use either a cleansing milk or cream. Complexion milks are suitable for removing normal make-up as they have a low oil content in an oil in water emulsion. For heavy make-up and stage make-up, a cleansing cream with a high oil content in the emulsion is more suitable.

The skin needs nourishing and certain emollient or nourishing creams are used. These act as a protective barrier over the face, protecting the skin against weather and dirt. Moisturizing creams are used as the skin begins to age, and the water content of the skin begins to lessen, causing dry skin. The main function of a moisturizing cream is to slow down the rate of evaporation of moisture in the skin. Moisturizing creams are very light and have a low oil content in comparison with nourishing creams, which have a high oil content.

4
Cream preparations

1 GENERAL PREPARATION; THE FORMATION OF EMULSIONS

An emulsion consists of two immiscible liquids, one being dispersed in the other. These are known as the internal and external phases respectively. Cosmetic emulsions are generally creams, examples of which can be found later in this chapter.

Most cosmetic emulsions are oil and water systems, of which there are two types. The type of emulsion obtained depends on the proportion of oil and water used. When the oil or fatty phase is dispersed in the aqueous or water phase, it is known as an oil in water (O/W) system. When the aqueous phase is dispersed in the oil phase it is referred to as a water in oil (W/O) system.

The two types of emulsions may be distinguished by several means. An oil in water emulsion is less greasy than a water in oil emulsion because water is the external phase. An oil in water emulsion is dispersible in water. It is also more easily washed than a water in oil emulsion, which is not so readily water dispersible. Again because water is the external phase, an oil in water emulsion will conduct electricity, whereas a water in oil emulsion will not conduct electricity unless an electrolyte has been added.

An emulsion of oil in water should consist of oil dispersed in the water. If a very small amount of oil is added to water it is comparatively easy to reduce it to very small droplets. Once in this state the droplets do not readily coalesce. This is due to electrical charges which form on the surfaces of the droplets. If a larger quantity of oil is required, it is less easy to mix with the water, and once mixed there is a tendency for the phases to separate. To prevent this an emulsifying agent is used. The emulsifying agent stabilizes the emulsion by forming a thin film over the droplets and preventing them from coalescing (Fig. 6).

Thus there are two main conditions which must be satisfied in the preparation of emulsions. The first is that the droplets of the internal phase must be small. This is ensured during the process of mixing, which should be designed to make the emulsion homogeneous throughout. Homogenizing the emulsion can be done by shaking the phases in a bottle, by stirring

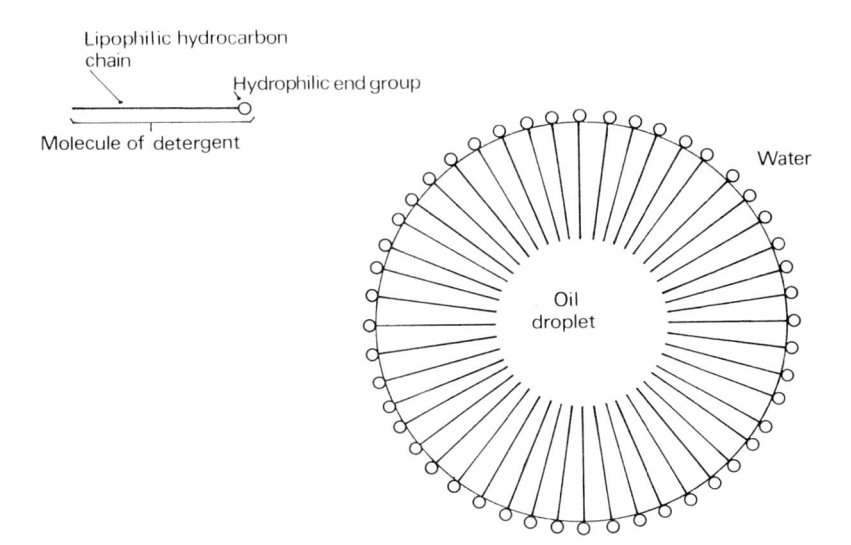

Fig. 6 Diagram of an oil droplet in an oil-in-water emulsion. The molecules of detergent are arranged so as to form a film around the oil droplet, thus preventing it from coalescing with other oil droplets.

them in a beaker or by using a mortar and pestle, depending usually on the nature of the oil phase. The second condition is that the droplets should have a thin film of emulsifying agent around them.

2 PREPARATION OF COSMETIC EMULSIONS

Note
1   All cosmetic emulsions should be prepared in glass containers. In the laboratory, glass beakers are the most suitable.
2   Care should be taken to follow the correct formula. This will ensure that the preparation is of the right consistency.

Ingredients

The Water Phase should contain all the water soluble materials such as glycerine and borax. All preparations must contain a preservative and an antioxidant. The proportion of water in a stable emulsion should not fall below 50% in any formula.

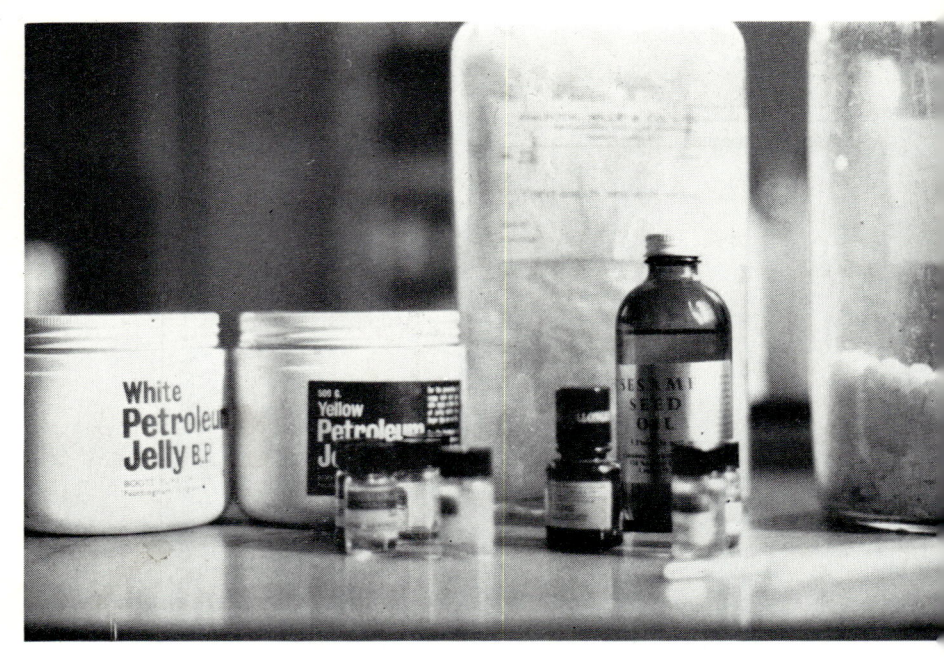

Fig. 7 Some ingredients of a cosmetic emulsion.

Some oil phase ingredients:

1   *Liquid paraffin:* This is one of the major oils used either as an ingredient in cleansing creams, or as a diluent for other fatty materials.

2   *Almond oil:* This is the best oil for cosmetic emulsions.

3   *Sesame oil:* This can be substituted for olive oil.

4   *Petroleum jelly:* This is sometimes used as an oil-thickening agent and emollient.

5   *Fatty acids—oleic acid:* This is the chief oil phase ingredient in vanishing and shaving creams.

6   *Esters:* Isopropyl myristate, isopropyl palmitate, isopropyl stearate—these are in liquid form and promote skin penetration.

7   *Spermaceti:* This is an excellent emollient.

8   *Carnauba wax:* This is the thickening agent for the oil phase.

9   *Beeswax:* This acts as an emollient and emulsifier.

Perfumes and insoluble powders are not added until after the phases have been mixed (see Method of Preparation).

The choice of an emulsifying agent: The first emulsifier to be used was soap, but nowadays oil soluble materials such as fatty alcohols (e.g. cetyl alcohol) and esters (e.g. glyceryl monostearate) are used. The choice of the emulsifying agent depends on two important factors:

1 The nature of the emulsion—that is, whether it is to be an oil in water or water in oil emulsion.

2 The compatibility of the emulsifying agent with the rest of the substances in the emulsion.

Most emulsifying agents produce oil in water systems. Some examples are wool-fats, beeswax-borax mixture, wool alcohols and triethanolamine. (Others may be found listed in Appendix II.)

If a *surfactant* (i.e. a surface active agent) is used to make oily or waxy substances mix with water, the resulting emulsion may be either opaque or clear. Many *detergents* are classed as surfactants and are often used to stabilize oil and water emulsions. A detergent molecule has a long hydrocarbon part which is insoluble in water but soluble in oil (hydrophobic and lipophilic). The ionic end group is insoluble in oil but soluble in water (hydrophilic and lipophobic). If a small amount of detergent is added to water, a colloidal suspension is formed. The hydrocarbon ends of the detergent molecules cluster together and leave their ionic end groups in contact with the water. If oil is then introduced and the whole stirred together, the hydrocarbon parts of the detergent molecules enter the oil droplets, leaving the ionic end groups in the water. Thus round the oil droplets is formed a film which is partly in the water and partly in the oil (see Fig. 6).

Method of preparation (See Fig. 8)

The phases. As most cosmetic emulsions are prepared from waxes and other substances that are normally solid at room temperature, the two phases must first be heated separately. The waxes and oils should be heated to about 10°C above the melting point of the highest melting wax, taking care not to overheat. This usually means heating the waxes to about 70°C. The water phase should be heated to a temperature 20°C above that of the oil phase, to allow for cooling when the phases are mixed.

Mixing and cooling. Generally the water phase should be

added to the oil phase. An exception to this is made in the case of high oil content (80–90%). There must be continuous stirring with a glass rod as there is a tendency for the phases to separate if stirring is stopped. The rate of cooling should be slow, to avoid coarsening of the emulsion. Stirring should continue until the temperature reaches about 40°C. Perfumes should be added whilst stirring, when the emulsion is partially cool (35°C). If there are any insoluble powders to be used in the preparation they should be heated to 75°C and added soon after the phases have been mixed.

Homogenizing. The finished preparation should be smooth and creamy. If this has not been achieved during the mixing

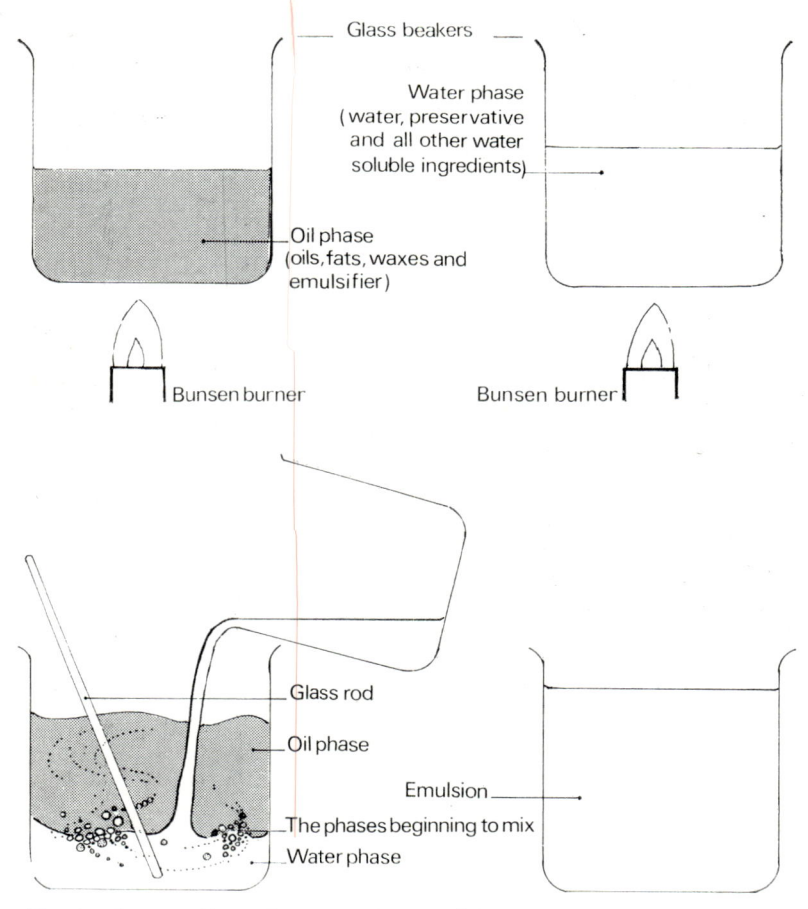

Fig. 8   Preparation of a cosmetic emulsion.

CREAM PREPARATIONS 27

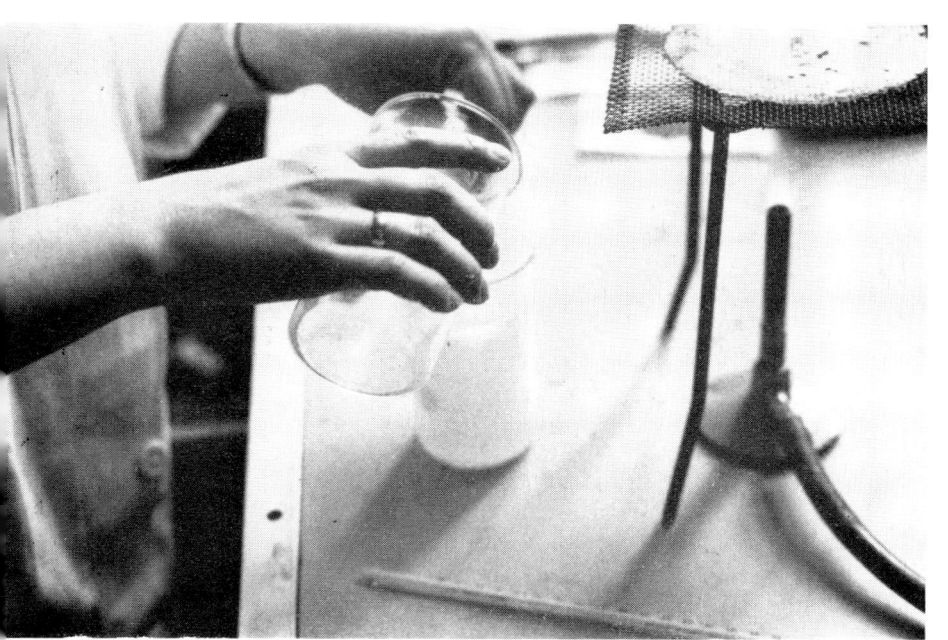

Fig. 8.1 Adding the water phase to the oil phase after heating to the required temperature.

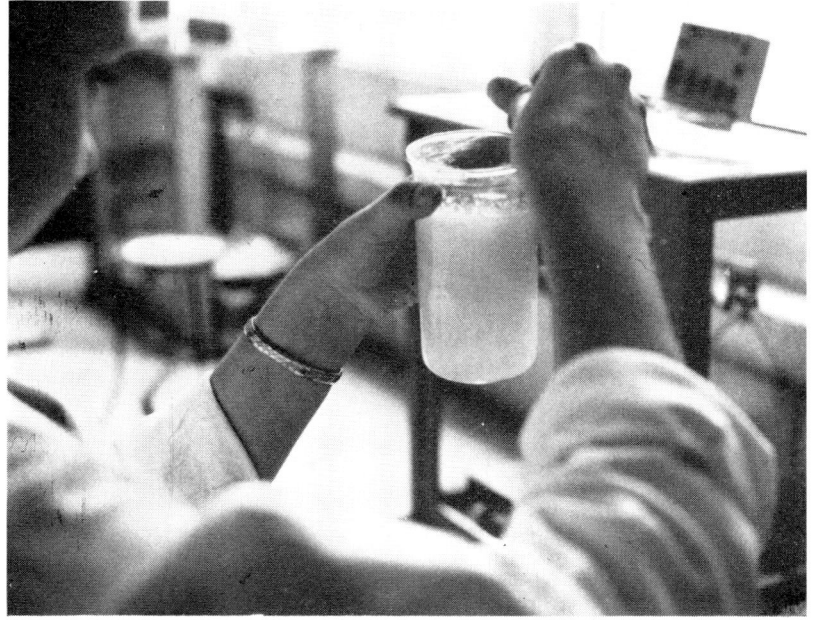

Fig. 8.2 Stirring and mixing the two phases immediately after they have been added together.

28 PRACTICAL COSMETIC SCIENCE

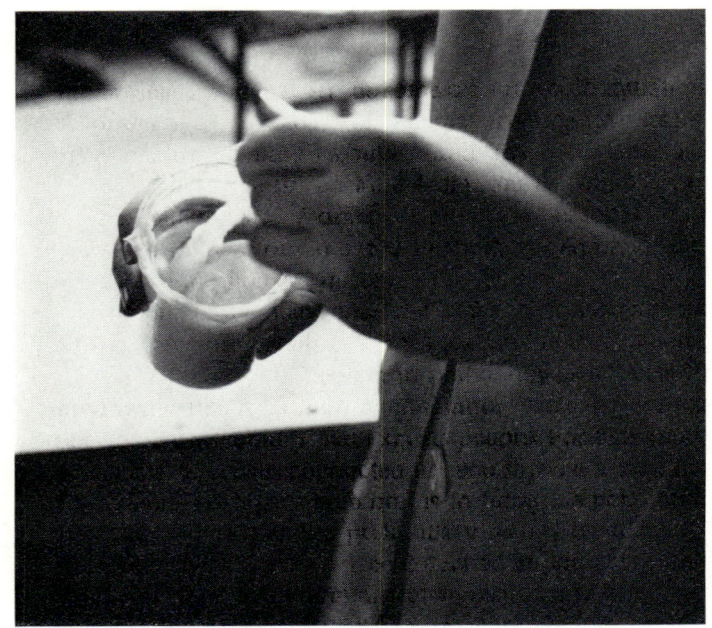

Fig. 8.3 The final stirring and mixing of the emulsion before checking the temperature prior to adding the perfume.

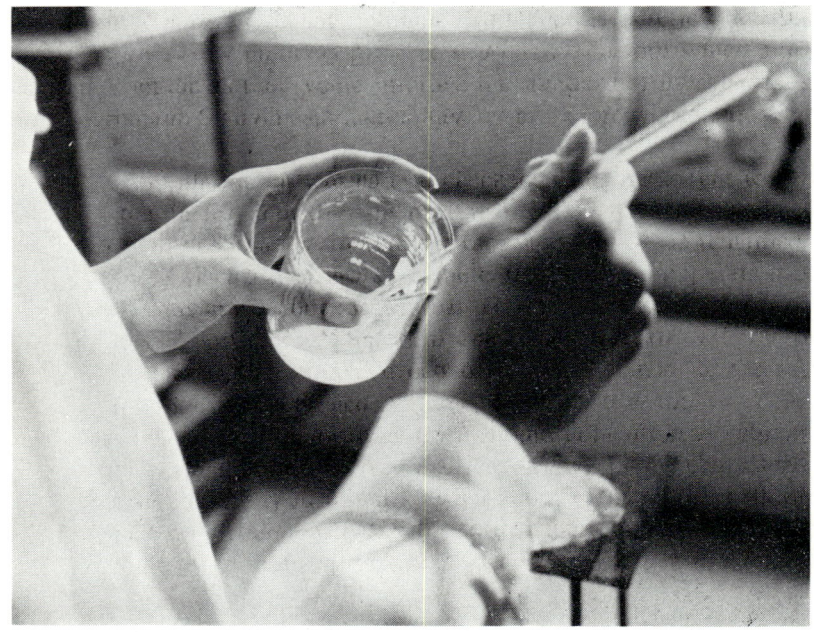

Fig. 8.4 Checking the temperature of the finished emulsion before adding the perfume (35°C).

CREAM PREPARATIONS   29

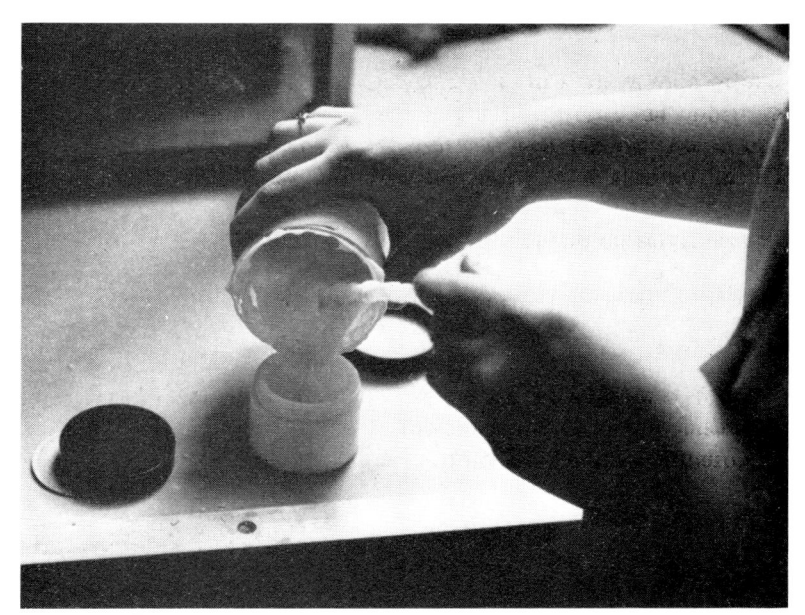

Fig. 8.5   Potting the cream.

process, it may be necessary to completely homogenize the emulsion at this stage. This may be done by using an ordinary whisk or, if the emulsion is semi-solid, by using a mortar and pestle. Homogenization helps to prepare a more stable emulsion by breaking up the drops of oil into smaller droplets (Fig. 9).

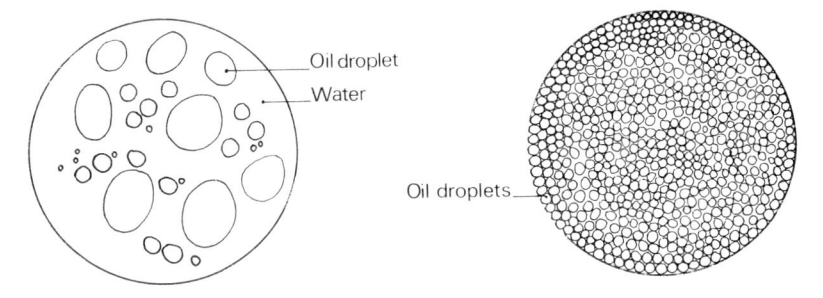

Fig. 9   Comparison of emulsions before and after homogenizing.

O/W emulsions. In preparing these emulsions it is best to make a preliminary mixture containing a portion of the water and emulsifier with an equal amount of oil. This should be stirred with a glass rod and homogenized slowly while the remaining oil is added. When the remaining water is added slowly to the oil phase, a very heavy W/O emulsion is formed. This will thin out suddenly to the O/W type of emulsion. When this happens the water can then be added more rapidly.

Control of the thickness of emulsions

Liquid emulsions tend to thicken. They then no longer pour. This increase in viscosity may be due to one or more of the following:

    1 too high a concentration of waxes in the oil phase
    2 too much emulsifying agent
    3 too much homogenizing.

To lower the viscosity of the emulsion any of the following methods may be used:

    1 Increase the proportion of the external phase.
    2 Decrease the proportion of the internal phase.
    3 Use a lower melting point ingredient in the internal phase.
    4 Add a water soluble emulsifier.

To raise the viscosity use one of the following methods:

    1 Increase the proportion of the internal phase.
    2 Add thickeners such as emulsifiers or gums.
    3 Include a higher melting point ingredient in the internal phase.

Causes of failure of emulsion preparations

1 Insufficient emulsifying agent. This is rarely the cause of trouble as the tendency is to add too much emulsifier.

2 Decomposition of the emulsifying agent. This could be due to chemical reaction or the activities of micro-organisms. The emulsifying agent may be destroyed by chemical reaction with one of the ingredients.

3 Temperature changes. An increase in temperature can cause the two phases to separate, if the emulsifier is susceptible to temperature variations. Freezing can also destroy an emulsion by the formation of ice crystals on the surface.

4 Presence of electrolytes. Occasionally, small quantities of electrolytes (e.g. calcium salts) are added to emulsions containing triethanolamine soaps. This causes the phases to separate.

5 The concentration of the phases. The concentration of the phases should be in the region of 60% water and 40% oil. A higher phase volume ratio than 60 : 40, i.e. too much water, tends to cause separation of the phases.

6 Rancidity of the oil. Some animal and vegetable oils may become rancid on prolonged storage and cause the phases to separate. Rancidity may be prevented by the addition of an antioxidant.

3 COLD/CLEANSING CREAMS

(a) Cold creams

Cold cream is an emulsion of water in oil. It possesses smoothness and sheen. It must not show separation of water in oil, shrinkage or specks. It must be neither too soft nor too stiff. It is called cold cream because of the cooling effect when applied to the skin, which is due to slow evaporation of the water in it. In place of mineral oil one can use almond oil, which nourishes the skin and cleanses it. Mineral oil, while not nourishing, cleanses and is much better for making the cream. It still gives the cold effect—hence cold/cleansing cream.

When any alkaline solution is added to an acid, neutralization will take place if the amounts of reacting substances are equal. When a fatty acid is the reacting agent, the neutralized product is called a soap. When stearic acid and sodium hydroxide react, the resulting products are sodium stearate (a soap) and water. If a hot solution of beeswax is neutralized with borax, as in cold cream, a similar set of reactions takes place.

The essential reaction is, therefore, neutralization of beeswax fatty acid producing a soap within the oily mass and simultaneously emulsifying fats in the water present. The resulting emulsion is of the oil in water type.

Some materials used in the preparation of cold/cleansing creams:

1 *Beeswax:* This gives body to the cream due to its free cerotic acid, and takes part in the emulsification.

2 *Paraffin wax, ozokerite, ceresine, etc:* All of these waxes give "body" (increase in density)) and smoothness.

3 *Mineral oil:* This promotes the cleansing action of the cream.

4 *Borax:* This substance is the alkali that reacts with the cerotic acid forming sodium cerolite, a soap, and causes the emulsification of the oil/water mixture.

5 *Spermaceti:* This gives a high gloss.

Formulae *Grammes*
1 a Mineral oil 28.0
    Isopropyl myristate 14.0
    Acetoglyceride L/C 2.5
    Petroleum jelly 7.5
    Beeswax 15.0
  b Borax 1.0
    Distilled water 32.0
    Preservative (Nipagin M) one microspatula-full
  c Perfume one or two drops

Method: Heat (*a*) and (*b*) to about 75°C in separate glass beakers. Add (*b*) to (*a*) slowly with continuous stirring, adding the perfume when the temperature has fallen to about 35°C.

2 a Beeswax 16.0
    Mineral oil 50.0
  b Borax 1.0
    Distilled water 33.0
    Preservative (Nipagin M) one microspatula-full
  c Perfume one or two drops

Method
1. Heat (*a*) and (*b*) to about 75°C in separate glass beakers.
2. Add (*b*) to (*a*). Stir slowly until the temperature drops to 50°C. Add perfume when the temperature has dropped to 35°C. Pour into jars.

3 a Beeswax 10.0
    Mineral oil 60.0
    Spermaceti 5.0
  b Borax 1.0
    Water 24.0
    Preservative (Nipagin M) one microspatula-full
  c Perfume one or two drops

Method: As above.

4 a Beeswax 12.0
    Almond oil 50.0
    Lanolin 0.5
  b Borax one microspatula-full
    Rose water 37.5
    Preservative (Nipagin M) one microspatula-full

   c Perfume   one or two drops
Method: As above.

5 *a* Beeswax   15.0
    Almond oil   55.0
 b Distilled water   29.0
    Borax   1.0
    Preservative (Nipagin M)   one microspatula-full
 c Perfume   one or two drops
Method: As above.

6 *a* Beeswax   10.0
    Mineral oil   50.0
    Paraffin wax   5.0
    Spermaceti   5.0
 b Distilled water   29.5
    Borax   0.5
    Preservative (Nipagin M)   one microspatula-full
 c Perfume   one or two drops
Method: As above.

7 *a* Beeswax   10.0
    Mineral oil   53.0
    Ceresine wax   5.0
    Spermaceti   3.0
 b Distilled water   28.4
    Borax   0.6
    Preservative (Nipagin M)   one microspatula-full
 c Perfume   one or two drops
Method: As above.

8 *a* Beeswax   9.0
    Ceresine wax   4.5
    Mineral oil   52.0
    Lanolin   0.5
 b Borax   0.7
    Distilled water   33.3
    Preservative (Nipagin M)   one microspatula-full
 c Perfume   one or two drops
Method: As above.

9 *a* Beeswax   14.5
    Almond oil   46.0
    Spermaceti   10.0
    Distilled water   29.5
 b Borax   one microspatula-full

Preservative (Nipagin M)	one microspatula-full
c Perfume	one or two drops

Method: As above.

10 a	Wheat-germ oil	48.0
	Spermaceti	15.0
	Beeswax	15.0
b	Distilled water	22.0
	Borax	one microspatula-full
	Preservative (Nipagin M)	one microspatula-full
c	Perfume	one to three drops

Method: As above.

11	Collone SE	10.0
	Distilled water	90.0
	Preservative (Nipagin M)	one microspatula-full
	Perfume	one drop

Method: Heat the mixture of collone SE, distilled water and preservative. When the collone has melted and a temperature of 75°C has been reached, stir the mixture, whilst cooling, until it thickens (50°C). Reheat until the mixture is smooth (approx. 70°C). Remove the heat source and continue stirring until the mixture has again thickened. Add the perfume at 50°C.

12	Collone SE	10.0
	Mineral oil	10.0
	Distilled water	80.0
	Preservative (Nipagin M)	one microspatula-full
	Perfume	one drop

Method: Dissolve the collone SE in the oil at 65°C. Add all the water at 80°C. Stir whilst cooling until the cream thickens. Add the perfume and preservative.

(b) Cleansing creams

Cleansing creams, as the name implies, are used to cleanse the skin and are used either instead of water, or prior to washing with water. Colouring materials used in make-up are more easily dissolved in such creams than in water, and so the use of an oily cream draws out the colour from the make-up and the impurities from the skin. The cleansing creams should leave the skin feeling smooth, immaculately clean and preferably non-greasy. Some cleansing creams are excellent for skins that become over-heated.

There are two types of cleansing creams:

1 Liquefying creams, consisting of oily materials (no water), and

2 Emulsified creams (water in oil).

The liquefying cleansing creams consist of mixtures of mineral oils or fatty materials, some hydrocarbon waxes, spermaceti, paraffin wax and cetyl alcohol, together with perfumes and preservatives.

The emulsified cleansing creams contain a great amount of water ranging from about 25% to 70%. They will also contain beeswax, mineral oils, stearic acid, lanolin, glycerine, perfumes and preservatives.

Cleansing milks are diluted cleansing creams and contain similar substances with the addition of triethanolamine. Cleansing lotions are useful in the treatment of greasy skins and consist of lotions such as sulphated olive oil and water to which may be added perfume and preservative.

Formulae *Grammes*

Liquefying cleansing creams
1   Mineral oil   80.0
    Petroleum jelly   15.0
    Ozokerite   5.0
    Perfume   one or two drops
    Preservative (Nipagin M)   one microspatula-full

Method: Heat all the oils and waxes together at 65°C. Cool with stirring. Add perfume and preservative at 45°C. Pour into jars.

2   Isopropyl myristate   25.0
    Mineral oil   25.0
    Petroleum jelly   30.0
    Paraffin wax   20.0
    Perfume   one or two drops
    Preservative (Nipagin M)   one microspatula-full

Method: As above.

3   White mineral oil   42.0
    White petroleum jelly   18.0
    Spermaceti   12.0
    Ozokerite   14.0
    Cetyl alcohol   14.0
    Perfume   one or two drops
    Preservative (Nipagin M)   one microspatula-full

Method: As above.

Emulsified cleansing creams

1
Mineral oil	30.0
Stearic acid	10.0
Triethanolamine	2.0
Sodium alginate	0.5
Distilled water	57.5
Perfume	one or two drops
Preservative (Nipagin M)	one microspatula-full

Method:
1. Mix the sodium alginate with the glycerine. Add the triethanolamine and water. Stir until the sodium alginate is dissolved.
2. Mix the stearic acid and mineral oil and heat to 70°C
3. Heat the water phase, (1), to 70°C. Add this to the oil phase, (2). Stir while cooling to 45°C. Add the perfume and preservative.

2
a	Mineral oil	40.0
	Ozokerite	3.0
	Cetyl alcohol	2.0
b	Sodium cetyl sulphate	1.0
	Water	54.0
c	Perfume	one or two drops
	Preservative (Nipagin M)	one microspatula-full

Method: Heat (*a*) to 70°C. Heat (*b*) to 70°C. Add (*b*) to (*a*) with slow stirring. Add the perfume and preservative at 50°C.

3
a	Mineral oil	40.0
	Paraffin wax	12.0
	Ozokerite	4.0
b	Sodium monolaurate	2.0
	Water	42.0
c	Perfume	one or two drops
	Preservative (Nipagin M)	one microspatula-full

Method: As above.

4
a	Beeswax	16.0
	Mineral oil	50.0
b	Borax	0.8
	Water	33.2
c	Perfume	one to three drops
d	Preservative (Nipagin M)	one microspatula-full

Method: Heat (*a*) to 75°C. Heat (*b*) to 75°C. Dissolve the preservative in (*b*). Add (*b*) to (*a*) with constant stirring. Add the perfume between 35°C and 45°C.

5 a Beeswax   11.5
     Spermaceti   2.6
     Carnauba wax   5.0
     Petroleum jelly   32.0
     Mineral oil   17.0
  b Borax   0.75
     Water   31.15
  c Perfume   one to three drops
     Preservatives (Nipagin M)   one microspatula-full

Method: As above.

Cleansing lotions
1   Triethanolamine lauryl sulphate
        liquid   5.0
    Water   95.0
    Perfume   one or two drops
    Preservative (Nipagin M)   one microspatula-full

Method: Mix the ingredients together and filter. Pour into bottles

2   Sulphated olive oil   10.0
    Water   90.0
    Perfume   one to three drops
    Preservative (Nipagin M)   one microspatula-full

Method: As above.

3   Triethanolamine lauryl sulphate
        liquid   5.0
    Propylene glycol *or* isopropyl
        myristate   10.0
    Water   85.0
    Perfume   one to three drops
    Preservative (Nipagin M)   one microspatula-full

Method: As above.

4   Toilet spirit   20.0
    Witch hazel   10.0
    Borax   1.0
    Water   69.0
    Perfume   three to five drops
    Preservative (Nipagin M)   one microspatula-full

Method: Dissolve the borax in water with the aid of gentle heat. Cool. Add the toilet spirit and witch hazel. Add the perfume and preservative and stir.

4 VANISHING/FOUNDATION CREAMS

(a) Vanishing creams

A vanishing cream is an emulsion of stearic acid. The external phase is water with an addition of oils, fats and other fatty acids. The emulsifying agent is soap or a mixture of soaps of sodium, potassium and ammonia. They are always oil in water emulsions.

They are called vanishing creams because they seem to disappear when rubbed into the skin. Sometimes they are called foundation creams as they form a foundation or base for powder. They can also be used as hand creams. The principal ingredients are:

1   *Stearic acid:* This forms the bulk of the oil phase which, by the addition of an alkali, forms a soap. Most of the stearic acid is emulsified by the soap formed. The balance remaining is very firmly dispersed through the whole cream.

2   *Cetyl alcohol:* This is obtained from China wax and is a waxy alcohol which, when added to an emulsion, makes the final product fine and smooth. It also gives added smoothness to the skin.

3   *Humectants:* Glycerine, sorbitol, etc., help to improve the spreading properties of the cream and preserve its consistency. They minimize the drying out of the cream on exposure to the air. The humectants are of three types—inorganic, organic and metal organic.

4   *Oils:* These are of vegetable origin, e.g. almond oil They nourish, protect and help to retain the suppleness of the skin.

5   *Alkalis:* These consist of sodium and/or potassium hydroxides, which cause the saponification of the stearic acid. It is better to use a hydroxide than a carbonate, because when stearic acid is added to a carbonate, it will not set free the carbon dioxide, which would remain in the finished cream. The cream would then have numerous minute bubbles rising to the surface, with the result that in time the cream would sink to the bottom of the jar.

6   *Triethanolamine:* This is a derivative of ammonia. It is supplied commercially as mono, di and triethanolamines. It is a viscous, colourless or faintly yellow liquid. It combines with fatty acids to form soaps. It is soluble in water, alcohol and chloroform.

Formulae

Grammes

1 *a* Stearic acid   5.0
    Lanette wax   15.0
  b Glycerine   7.0
    Distilled water   73.0
    Preservative (Nipagin M)   one microspatula-full
  c Perfume   one drop

Method: Heat part (*a*) to 70°C. Heat part (*b*) to 70°C. Add (*b*) to (*a*) with continuous stirring. Add perfume when cooled down to 35°C. (As the emulsion begins to cool it may appear to separate or curdle, but with continuous stirring it will become homogeneous again.)

2 *a* Lanette wax   5.0
    Stearic acid   15.0
  b Glycerine   7.0
    Distilled water   73.0
    Preservative (Nipagin M)   one microspatula
  c Perfume   one drop

Method: As above. (This forms a thicker cream.)

3 *a* Acetoglyceride S/C/4   2.0
    Stearic acid   18.0
  b Glycerine   5.0
    Potassium hydroxide   1.0
    Distilled water   74.0
    Preservative (Nipagin M)   one microspatula-full
  c Perfume   one drop

Method: Heat (*a*) in a beaker to 75°C. Heat (*b*) in a beaker to 75°C. Add (*b*) to (*a*) stirring continuously. Cool down to 45°C. Add perfume.

4 *a* Abracol GMS   12.0
    Liquid paraffin   2.0
    Spermaceti   5.0
  b Glycerine   3.0
    Distilled water   78.0
    Preservative (Nipagin M)   one microspatula-full
  c Perfume   one drop

Method: As above.

5 *a* Stearic acid   20.0
    Cetyl alcohol   0.50
    Triethanolamine   1.20
  b Sodium hydroxide   0.36
    Glycerine   8.0

		Distilled water	69.94
		Preservative (Nipagin M)	one microspatula-full
	c	Perfume	three or four drops

Method: As above.

6	a	Lanolin	2.0
		Cetyl alcohol	0.50
		Stearic acid	10.0
		Propylene glycol	8.0
		Potassium hydroxide	one microspatula-full
	b	Distilled water	79.50
		Preservative (Nipagin M)	one microspatula-full
	c	Perfume	three or four drops

Method: As above.

7	a	Stearic acid	12.0
		Cetyl alcohol	0.5
		Sorbitol syrup	5.0
		Isopropyl myristate	
		or propylene glycol	3.0
		Triethanolamine	1.0
	b	Glycerine	0.3
		Distilled water	78.2
		Preservative (Nipagin M)	one microspatula-full
	c	Perfume	three or four drops

Method: As above.

8	a	Stearic acid	25.0
		Spermaceti	5.0
	b	Distilled water	60.5
		Glycerol	8.0
		Preservative (Nipagin M)	one microspatula-full
	c	Perfume	one or two drops

Method: As above.

9	a	Stearic acid	15.0
		Potassium hydroxide	0.50
		Sodium hydroxide	0.18
		Cetyl alcohol	0.50
		Isopropyl myristate	3.0
	b	Glycerine	5.0
		Distilled water	75.82
		Preservative (Nipagin M)	one microspatula-full
	c	Perfume	one or two drops

Method: As above.

CREAM PREPARATIONS

10 *a*	Isopropyl myristate	2.0
	Stearic acid	18.0
	Cetyl alcohol	0.5
b	Potassium hydroxide	1.0
	Glycerine	8.0
	Distilled water	70.5
	Preservative (Nipagin M)	one microspatula-full
c	Perfume	three or four drops

Method: As above.

11 *a*	Lanette wax SX	8.0
b	Cetyl alcohol	5.0
c	Stearic acid	8.0
d	Glycerine	6.0
e	Titanium dioxide	2.0
f	Distilled water	70.0
g	Preservative (Nipagin M)	one microspatula-full
h	Perfume	two drops

Method:
1 Heat (*a*), (*b*) and (*c*) together to 75°C. Mix the titanium dioxide with the glycerine in a mortar and add this mixture to the melted waxes.
2 Dissolve the preservative in the water (75°C). Add (2) to (1) and stir until the mixture thickens. Add the perfume.

(b) Foundation creams

These are applied after cleansing. They must spread well and possess holding power for powder. There are two types:

1 pigmented creams which are coloured (the pigments must be carefully blended into the cream), and

2 unpigmented creams which can be used either as a foundation for powder, or simply as a vanishing cream.

Formulae   *Grammes*

1 *a*	Glycerine monostearate (self-emulsifying wax)	16.0
	Distilled water	44.0
	Preservative (Nipagin M)	one microspatula-full
b	Glycerine	25.0
	Powder base	15.0
	Colour	one microspatula-full
	Perfume	one or two drops

Method: Heat (*a*) to 85°–90°C. Mix the colour and perfume with the powder base (see chapter for making base), then disperse this in the glycerine. Add (*b*) to (*a*) and mix thoroughly.

2 a Lanette wax   8.0
     Stearic acid   8.0
     Distilled water   64.0
     Preservative (Nipagin M)   one microspatula-full
  b Glycerine   10.0
     Powder base   10.0
     Colour   one microspatula-full
     Perfume   three or four drops

Method: As above.

3 a Acetoglyceride L/C   10.0
     Acetoglyceride S/C/2   10.0
     Mineral oil (liquid paraffin
       —cosmetic quality)   5.0
     Stearic acid   5.0
  b Glycerine   5.0
     Triethanolamine   0.5
     Distilled water   64.5
     Preservative (Nipagin M)   one microspatula-full
  c Perfume   three or four drops

Method: Heat (*a*) and (*b*) independently to 75°C. Add (*b*) to (*a*) slowly with continuous stirring. Cool with stirring, adding the perfume at about 35°C. Lake colours can be added if desired.

4 a Spermaceti   5.0
     Glycerine   5.0
     Glycerine monostearate   20.0
     Colours   3.0
  b Distilled water   67.0
     Preservative (Nipagin M)   one microspatula-full
  c Perfume   three or four drops

Method: Heat (*a*) to about 75°C. with constant stirring to disperse the colours. Stir until the consistency is smooth. Re-heat to 75°C. Heat (*b*) to 75°C. Add (*b*) to (*a*). Cool with stirring. Add the perfume at 35°C.

5   Isopropyl myristate   20.0
     Petroleum jelly   55.0
     Titanium dioxide   10.0
     Kaolin   15.0
     Preservative (Nipagin M)   one microspatula-full
     Colours   one microspatula-full
     Perfume   three or four drops

Method: Prepare a smooth paste of the colours, titanium dioxide and kaolin with the Isopropyl myristate. Warm gently. Heat petroleum jelly to 70°C. Add to the first part. Mix together thoroughly.

6 a	Lanette wax SX	13.0
	Lanolin	1.0
	Lecithin	0.5
	Cetyl alcohol	10.0
	Isopropyl alcohol	7.5
b	Distilled water	66.0
	Preservative (Nipagin M)	one microspatula-full
c	Grapefruit juice *or* lemon juice	2.0
d	Perfume	three drops

Method: Heat (*a*) and (*b*) independently to 75°C. Add (*b*) to (*a*). Add the fruit juice after cooling down to 45°C. Then add the perfume.

7 a	Castor oil	2.0
	Stearic acid	5.0
	Cetyl alcohol	2.0
b	Glycerine	5.0
	Borax	1.0
	Sodium hydroxide	one microspatula-full
	Preservative (Nipagin M)	one microspatula-full
	Distilled water	85.0
c	Perfume	three drops

Method: Heat (*a*) and (*b*) independently to 70°C. Add (*b*) to (*a*). Cool with stirring to 35°C. Add the perfume.

8 a	Lanette wax	16.0
	Almond oil *or* Olive oil	6.0
b	Glycerine	7.0
	Citric acid *or* lemon juice	0.3
	Distilled water	70.7
	Preservative (Nipagin M)	one microspatula-full
c	Perfume	three drops

Method: As above.

9 a	Lanette wax SX	16.0
	Lanolin	3.0
	Lecithin	1.0
b	Glycerine	7.0
	Citric acid *or* lemon juice	1.0
	Distilled water	72.0
	Preservative (Nipagin M)	one microspatula-full
c	Perfume	three drops

5 NOURISHING CREAMS AND SKIN FOODS

Method: As above.
    (N.B. The perfume can be omitted if not required)

Formulae *Grammes*

1 *Dry Skin Cream*
   a Sunflower oil 5.5
      Isopropyl linoleate 1.0
      Cetyl alcohol 2.0
      Abracol GMS (Emulsifier) 12.5
   b Almond oil 8.0
      Distilled water 71.0
      Preservative (Nipagin M) one microspatula-full
   c Perfume three drops

Method: Heat (a) and (b) independently to about 75°C. Add (b) to (a) with stirring. Add the perfume when cool (35°).

2 *Moisturizing Cream*
   a Soya bean oil 7.5
      Cetyl alcohol 2.0
      Isopropyl linoleate 1.0
      Polyethylene glycol
        monostearate 12.5
      Abracol GMS (emulsifier) 7.5
   b Distilled water 61.3
      Sodium lauryl sulphate 1.2
      Glycerine 8.0
      Preservative (Nipagin M) one microspatula-full
   c Perfume three drops

Method: As above.

3 *Moisturizing Cream*
   a Glyceryl monostearate 14.0
      Lanolin 2.0
      Cetyl alcohol 2.0
      Spermaceti 5.0
      Almond oil 8.0
      Olive oil 8.0
      Glycerine 5.0
   b Distilled water 56.0
      Preservative (Nipagin M) one microspatula-full
      Antioxidant (Progallin) one drop
   c Perfume three drops

Method: As above.

4   *Nourishing Milk*
   a Glyceryl laurate   10.0
     Carotene oil   1.5
     Wheat germ oil   5.0
   b Distilled water   83.5
     Preservative (Nipagin M) one microspatula-full
   c Perfume   three drops

Method: As above.

5   *Liquid Skin Food (for dry skin)*
   a Toilet spirit   5.0
     Wheat germ oil   5.0
     Ethylene glycol stearate 3.0
     Sunflower oil   10.0
     Cholesterol   one microspatula-full
     Lecithin   one microspatula-full
   b Distilled water   77.0
     Preservative (Nipagin M) one microspatula-full
   c Perfume   five drops

Method: Dissolve lecithin and cholesterol in the toilet spirit. Add other ingredients under (*a*). Heat (*a*) and (*b*) independently to 70°–75°C. Add (*b*) to (*a*). Add perfume at 35°C.

6   *Cleansing and Nourishing Milk*
   a Isopropyl palmitate   1.0
     Almond oil   1.5
     Wheat germ oil   1.5
     Glycol laurate   15.0
     Glyceryl stearate   3.5
   b Rose water   77.5
     Preservative (Nipagin M) one microspatula-full
   c Perfume   three drops

Method: Heat (*a*) and (*b*) independently to 75°C. Add (*b*) to (*a*) with stirring. Add the perfume.

7   *Honey Milk*
   a Almond or peanut oil, or any
       vegetable oil   2.0
     Glycol stearate   7.0
     Cetyl alcohol   1.5
   b Distilled water   87.5
     Preservative (Nipagin M) one microspatula-full
   c Perfume   three drops
   d Honey   2.0

Method: Heat (*a*) and (*b*) independently to 75°C. Add (*b*) to (*a*). Add the perfume at 35°C. Stir in the honey.

8   Dry Skin Lotion
    Cholesterol   0.05
    Lecithin   0.05
    Toilet Spirit   5.0
    Ethylene glycol stearate   3.0
    Linseed, ground nut
      or avocado oil   10.0
    Glycerine   5.0
    Distilled water   76.0
    Preservative (Nipagin M)   one microspatula-full
    Perfume   one or two drops

Method:
1 Dissolve lecithin and cholesterol in the toilet spirit. Heat the oils and the ethylene glycol stearate.
2 Mix the glycerine, preservative and water and heat to 70°C. Add (2) to (1). Add the perfume.

9   Lemon Juice Cream
    a Lanette wax   12.0
    b Myristyl alcohol   5.0
    c Glycerine   6.0
    d Lemon juice   20.0
    e Oil of lemon   one or two drops
    f Preservative (Nipagin M) one microspatula-full
    g Distilled water   57.0

Method:
1 Heat (a) and (b) to 75°C.
2 Heat (g) and (f) to 75°C. Add (2) to (1). Stir in the lemon juice after the emulsion has formed, then add the oil of lemon.

10 Fruit Juice Cream
    a Emulsene   16.0
       Sunflower oil   5.0
       Glycerine   5.0
       Orange juice or grapefruit
         juice   24.0
    b Distilled water   50.0
       Perfume (or orange oil
         if required)   one drop
       Preservative (Nipagin M) one microspatula-full

Method: Heat (a) to 75°C (with the exception of juice). Heat water and preservative to 75°C. Add (b) to (a). Stir in the juice after the emulsion has formed.

6 ASTRINGENT LOTIONS AND SKIN TONICS

These are used for the correction of an oily or dry skin. Astringent lotions have a mildly anti-perspirant action. In general they contain aluminium salts such as potassium aluminium sulphate, the salts of zinc such as zinc sulphate or phenosulphate, a small amount of alcohol (which gives a cooling effect), some camphor water, witch hazel, tincture of benzoin and perfumes or aromatic waters such as rose or orange flower waters. Skin tonics are not really tonics at all, but skin fresheners. They consist of diluted astringent lotions or can be based on alcohol with witch hazel and other ingredients such as fruit juices, borax, herbal extracts and infusions. Skin-food creams act as lubricants. They do not nourish the skin. Their main function is to delay the rate at which moisture is lost from the skin and so help to delay the ageing of the skin by keeping the outer layer soft and supple. They can also help to prevent wrinkles and lines in the skin for a certain time only. They do not prevent the ultimate occurrence of wrinkles.

The most important ingredient in a so called skin-food is lanolin, as it is very similar to sebum, which is the natural skin lubricant. Other lubricants which can be put into a skin food are wheat germ oil (this can be purchased from any health food store), cod liver oil, corn oil, avocado oil, sunflower oil, other suitable vegetable oils and mineral oil.

Formulae *Grammes*

1	Zinc sulphate	0.3
	Glycerine	5.0
	Potassium aluminium sulphate	1.0
	Rose water	50.0
	Distilled water	43.7
	Preservative (Nipagin M)	one microspatula-full

Method:
1. Dissolve the preservative and aluminium or zinc salts in distilled water by heating.
2. Cool the solution.
3. Add the rose water or orange flower water.
4. Place in a refrigerator for one week.
5. Filter.

2	Glycerine	6.0
	Orange-flower water	35.0

Rose-water	35.0
Potassium aluminium sulphate	4.0
Distilled water	20.0
Preservative (Nipagin M)	one microspatula-full
Colour (if required)	one microspatula-full

Method: As above.

Acne Preparations

1
Triethanolamine lauryl sulphate	80.0
Salicylic acid	2.5
Precipitated sulphur	0.5
Toilet spirit	0.5
Lavender oil	0.5
Rose water	6.5
Glycerine	5.0
Preservative (Nipagin M)	one microspatula-full

Method: Thoroughly mix all the ingredients. Do not cork for about half an hour after mixing to allow the excess of gas (which the solution cannot dissolve) to escape. This solution must be used immediately, as it becomes valueless if kept too long.

2
Precipitated sulphur	10.0
Glycerine	10.0
Spirit of camphor	10.0
Distilled water	70.0
Preservative (Nipagin M)	one microspatula-full

Method: Mix the sulphur with the glycerine. Add the spirit of camphor. Then add the distilled water and preservative, and mix thoroughly. Filter.

Special Creams for Very Greasy Skin

1
a Petroleum jelly	5.0
b Isopropyl linoleate	2.0
c Lanolin	5.0
d Isopropyl myristate	5.0
e Cetyl alcohol	12.0
f Cetrimide	1.0
g Glycerine	15.0
h Zinc oxide	25.0
i Distilled water	30.0
j Abracol LDS	one microspatula-full
k Preservative (Nipagin M)	one microspatula-full

Method:
1. Heat (a) (b) (c) (d) and (e) (75°C).
2. Incorporate the zinc oxide (h).
3. Warm (f) (g) (i) and (k) to 45°C. Add to other ingredients. Stir.

2 The following cream has a low total oil content and can be used sparingly as a foundation cream, or for the treatment of greasy conditions of the skin or scalp.

a	Isopropyl myristate	3.0
b	Isopropyl palmitate	2.5
c	Cetyl alcohol	5.0
d	Glycerine	5.0
e	Distilled water	84.5
f	Preservative (Nipagin M)	one microspatula-full

Method: Heat (a) (b) and (c) together (75°C). Add (d) and (f) to (e) and warm (45°C). Add to the other ingredients. Stir.

3 A similar cream with a higher total oil phase.

a	Isopropyl myristate	6.0
b	Isopropyl palmitate	4.0
c	Cetyl alcohol	4.5
d	Lanolin	2.0
e	Glycerine	5.0
f	Distilled water	78.5
g	Preservative (Nipagin M)	one microspatula-full

Method: Heat (a) (b) (c) and (d) together (75°C). Add (e) and (g) to (f) and warm (45°C). Add to the other ingredients. Stir.

7 HAND CLEANING CREAMS

Hand cleaning creams are very useful in schools, factories or households. They are used a great deal in engineering factories and motor car industries for the easy removal of oil, dirt, grease, etc. The creams vary from liquids to transparent jellies, from stiff creams to mobile types of creams. The basic ingredients are very similar; they all contain a solvent, kerosene, as an oil in water emulsion.

To stabilize the emulsion, balance emulsifiers and surface active agents are added. When this cream or jelly is rubbed into the hands, the emulsion breaks down, liquefies and releases the oil and water to clean off the grease, oil or dirt. The emulsion breaks down because of the rapid evaporation of the water phase which destroys the phase volume ratio.

Formulae   *Grammes*

1   *Cream Type (stiff)*

a	Mineral oil (liquid paraffin)	29.0
	Empilan CDE	10.0
	Kerosene	1.0
	Stearic acid	9.0
	Glycerine	1.0
b	Distilled water	50.0
	Preservative (Nipagin M)	one microspatula-full

Method: Heat (*a*) and (*b*) independently to 70°C. Add (*b*) to (*a*). Stir until a mobile cream is produced. Cool with constant stirring.

Note: Perfume may be added to the emulsions, but this type of cream is not usually perfumed.

2 *Jelly Type*

a	Kerosene	20.0
	Empilan CDE	12.0
	Empicol LZ	0.5
	Oleic acid	2.0
b	Sodium hydroxide	0.25
	Distilled water	65.0
	Preservative (Nipagin M)	one microspatula-full

Method: Heat (*a*) and (*b*) independently to 70°C. Stir until homogeneous. Add (*b*) to (*a*). Stir and cool.

3

Neutral sulphated castor oil	97.0
Pure castor oil	1.0
Detergent (turkey red oil)	2.0
Perfume	one drop
Preservative (Nipagin M)	one microspatula-full

Method: Mix the oils together by heating (70°C). Add the perfume and preservative.

4 *Barrier Cream*

a	Empilan GMS	14.0
	Beeswax	4.0
	Lanolin	6.0
	Stearyl alcohol	2.0
	Empilan LZ	1.0
b	Zinc stearate	15.0
	Glycerine	4.0
	Distilled water	54.0
	Preservative (Nipagin M)	one microspatula-full

Method: Heat (*a*) in a beaker to 70°–75°C. Dissolve the preservative in water with the aid of gentle heat (35°C). Mix the zinc stearate with the glycerine. Add the water a little at a time. Then add (*b*) to (*a*) and stir until an emulsion is formed.

5 Barrier Cream
  a Empilan GMS SE32   12.0
     White petroleum jelly   3.0
     Beeswax   5.0
  b Glycerine   5.0
     Distilled water   65.0
  c Talc   10.0
  d Preservative (Nipagin M) one microspatula-full
     Perfume   one drop

Method: Heat (*a*) and (*b*) independently to 70°C. Stir (*c*) into (*b*) and (*b*) to (*a*). Add (*d*).

6 a Lanette wax SX   20.0
     Liquid paraffin   5.0
     Paraffin wax   5.0
  b Distilled water   70.0
     Preservative (Nipagin M) one microspatula-full

Method: Heat (*a*) and (*b*) independently to 60°–70°C. Pour (*b*) into (*a*) with continuous stirring.

Note: As the emulsion begins to cool, it may appear to separate or curdle, but under continuous stirring it becomes homogeneous again and will remain so when cool.

8 HAND CREAMS

These must provide a source of moisture to hands which are constantly exposed to soap, water and detergents. They should also provide some form of oil and leave the hands feeling soft but not very greasy. Hand cosmetics consist of lotions, emulsions, jellies, and mixtures of oil and water.

Formulae   *Grammes*

Hand Creams
1 a Mineral oil   3.0
     Lanolin   3.0
     Glycerol monostearate 12.0
  b Distilled water   77.0
     Sorbitol solution   5.0
     Preservative (Nipagin M) one microspatula-full
  c Perfume   one to three drops

Method: Heat (*a*) to 75°C. Heat (*b*) to 70°C. Add (*b*) to (*a*) with constant stirring. Cool to 35°C. Add the perfume.

2 a Isopropyl linoleate   1.0
     Acetoglyceride L/C   2.5
     Isopropyl myristate   5.0

Ethylene glycol monostearate	0.5
Emulsene 1220 (emulsifier)	2.5
b Distilled water	88.5
Preservative (Nipagin M)	one microspatula-full
c Perfume	one to three drops

Method: Heat (a) and (b) independently to about 75°C and add (b) to (a) slowly with continuous stirring. Add the perfume when the temperature has fallen to about 35°C.

Notes:

Isopropyl linoleate is readily absorbed by the skin. It is an emollient and has healing properties of value in products intended for dry skin conditions.

Ethylene glycol monostearate: On warming, it dissolves in most organic solvents including aromatic and halogenated hydrocarbons, esters, ketones, vegetable oils and higher alcohols. It is partly soluble in mineral oil, but is virtually insoluble in glycerine, propylene glycol, methanol and water. It has excellent stability and retains its good initial colour and odour on prolonged storage.

3 a Abracol LDS	5.0
Ethylene glycol monostearate	5.0
Mineral oil (cosmetic quality)	10.0
b Glycerine	5.0
Distilled water	75.0
Preservative (Nipagin M)	one microspatula-full
c Perfume	one to three drops

Method: as above.

4 a Abracol LDS	5.0
Ethylene glycol monostearate	5.0
Mineral oil (cosmetic quality)	10.0
Isopropyl palmitate	10.0
b Glycerine	2.0
Distilled water	68.0
Preservative (Nipagin M)	one microspatula-full
c Perfume	one to three drops

Method: As above.

5 a Abracol LDS	10.0
Isopropyl palmitate stearate	2.5

	Cetyl alcohol	2.0
	Mineral oil	12.5
	Lanolin anhydrous	2.0
	Stearic acid	8.0
b	Glycerine	10.0
	Distilled water	53.0
	Preservative (Nipagin M)	one microspatula-full
c	Perfume	one to three drops

Method: as above.

6 a	Collone SE	6.0
	Cetyl alcohol	2.0
	Liquid paraffin	25.0
	Glycerine	17.0
b	Distilled water	40.0
	Witch hazel	10.0
c	Perfume	one to three drops
	Preservative (Nipagin M)	one microspatula-full

Method: Heat (*a*) to 70°C. Dissolve the witch hazel in the water, heat to 75°C. Add (*b*) to (*a*), stir, cool down to 35°C. Add the perfume and preservative.

Hand Creams using Empilan

7 a	Empilan GMS	10.0
	Cetyl alcohol	1.0
	Stearic acid	5.0
b	Glycerine	7.5
	Titanium dioxide	1.0
	Distilled water	75.5
	Preservative (Nipagin M)	one microspatula-full
c	Perfume	three drops

Method: Mix the titanium oxide with the glycerine in a mortar. Heat (*a*) and (*b*) independently to about 75°C and add (*b*) to (*a*) slowly with continuous stirring. 35°C.

8 a	Empilan GMS	8.0
	Cetyl alcohol	1.0
	Stearic acid	5.0
b	Glycerine	12.0
	Titanium dioxide	1.0
	Distilled water	72.0
	Preservative (Nipagin M)	one microspatula-full
c	Perfume	three drops

Method: As above.

Hand Lotions

1 a	Cetyl alcohol	1.0

	Fluilan (liquid lanolin)	1.0
	Stearic acid	3.0
	MS/200/10 Silicone	0.25
b	Glycerine	2.0
	Triethanolamine	0.75
	Distilled water	92.0
c	Perfume	three drops
	Preservative (Nipagin M)	one microspatula-full

Method: Heat (*a*) and (*b*) independently to 70°C. Add (*b*) to (*a*). Cool to 40°C. Add the perfume and preservative.

2 a	Cetyl alcohol	0.50
	Fluilan	1.0
	Stearic acid	3.0
	MS/200/10 Silicone	1.0
b	Glycerine	2.0
	Triethanolamine	0.75
	Distilled water	91.25
c	Perfume	three drops
	Preservative (Nipagin M)	one microspatula-full

Method: As above.

3 a	Emulsifier (cetyl alcohol or Abracol LDS)	10.0
	Spermaceti	3.0
	Vegetable oil	6.0
	Stearic acid	5.0
	Oil of calendula (from marigold plant)	4.0
	Vitamin F	2.0
b	Distilled water	61.9
	Sorbitol solution	8.0
c	Perfume	three or four drops
	Preservative (Nipagin M)	one microspatula-full

Method: As above.

4 a	Isopropyl myristate	5.0
	Acetoglyceride L/C	2.5
	Diethylene glycol monostearate	0.5
	Cetyl alcohol	0.5
b	Distilled water	91.5
c	Perfume	three drops
	Preservative (Nipagin M)	one microspatula-full

Method: As above.

5 a Isopropyl myristate   5.0
    Mineral oil   2.0
    Acetoglyceride L/C   2.0
    Stearic acid   3.0
    Lanette wax   0.25
    Triethanolamine   1.0
  b Distilled water   86.75
  c Perfume   three drops
    Preservative (Nipagin M)   one microspatula-full

Method: As above.

6 a Petroleum jelly   10.0
    Cetyl alcohol   5.0
    Acetoglyceride S/C   5.0
    Acetoglyceride L/C   2.5
    Triethanolamine glyceryl
      monostearate   one microspatula-full
  b Distilled water   77.5
  c Perfume   three drops
    Preservative (Nipagin M)   one microspatula-full

Method: As above.

9 SUNSCREEN OILS AND CREAMS

Small doses of sunlight are very beneficial to the skin, but if the skin is over-exposed to the sun, burning of the skin can take place, and if the exposure is excessive, cancer of the skin may occur. To avoid burning, but to allow the skin to become tanned, certain substances can be incorporated into a formula. This permits the absorption of the harmful rays of the sun at the same time allowing the ultraviolet rays to act upon the melanin pigments, the amount of which is increased. These migrate from the lower layers to the surface of the skin and cause the skin to have a tanned appearance.

Formulae   *Grammes*

1   *Sunscreen Oil Base*
    Isopropyl myristate   10.0
    Antiviray   10.0
    Mineral oil (cosmetic
      quality)   80.0
    Perfume   one drop
    Colour   one drop
    Preservative (Nipagin M)   one microspatula-full

Method: Dissolve the perfume and preservative in the isopropyl myristate. Stir in the antiviray, then the mineral oil. Add the colour and stir well.

Note: Antiviray is a pale coloured liquid, an oil-soluble sun-screening agent especially prepared for use in anti-sunburn creams, lotions, oils and aerosol sprays. In general, between 5% and 10% of antiviray should be used. In most cases 8% gives adequate protection. It is soluble in ethyl alcohol and in mineral and vegetable oils.

2   *Sunscreen Oil Base*

Isopropyl myristate	90.0
Antiviray	10.0
Perfume	one drop
Colour	one drop
Preservative (Nipagin M)	one microspatula-full

Method: Mix the perfume, preservative and colour with the isopropyl myristate. Add the antiviray. Stir well.

3   *Sunscreen Cream Base*

a	Antiviray	8.0
	Stearic acid	1.7
	Isopropyl myristate	6.0
	Abracol PGS	3.5
b	Triethanolamine	0.8
	Distilled water	80.0
	Preservative (Nipagin)	one microspula-full
c	Perfume	one drop

Method: Heat (a) and (b) independently to about 75°C and add (b) to (a) slowly with continuous stirring. Cool with stirring, adding the perfume when the temperature has fallen to about 35°C.

4   *Sunscreen Cream*

Polychol 5	1.0
Volpo No. 3	3.0
Mineral oil	4.0
Squalene	8.0
Antiviray	2.0
Glycerine	4.0
Distilled water	78.0
Preservative (Nipagin M)	one microspatula-full

Method: Dissolve the polychol 5 in the volpo No. 3, mineral oil, glycerine, squalene and antiviray. Cool to room temperature. Add the water and preservative to the oils with stirring. No heat required.

5 Sunscreen Cream

a	Acetoglyceride L/C	5.0
	Antiviray	8.0
	Isopropyl myristate	15.0
	Cetyl alcohol	2.5
	Abracol GMS (emulsifier)	13.0
b	Sodium lauryl sulphate paste	0.1
	Propylene glycol	8.0
	Distilled water	48.4
	Preservative (Nipagin M)	one microspatula-full
c	Perfume	one or two drops

Method: Heat (a) and (b) independently to about 75°C and add (b) to (a) slowly with continuous stirring, adding the perfume when the temperature has fallen to about 35°C.

6 Sunscreen Lotion

Isopropyl myristate	10.0
Toilet spirit	80.0
Antiviray	10.0
Perfume	one or two drops
Colour (spirit soluble)	one drop

Method: Dissolve the antiviray in the isopropyl myristate. Then add this mixture to the toilet spirit. Add the perfume.

7 Sunscreen Lotion

Isopropyl myristate	2.0
Antiviray	10.0
Toilet spirit	88.0
Perfume	one or two drops
Colour (spirit soluble)	one drop

Method: As above.

8 Sunscreen Lotion (*Emulsion*)

a	Antiviray	10.0
	Ethylene glycol monostearate	2.0
	Emulsene 1220 (emulsifier)	2.5
b	Glycerine	8.0
	Distilled water	77.5
	Preservative (Nipagin M)	one microspatula-full
c	Perfume	one or two drops
d	Colour (water soluble) (if required)	one drop

Method: Dissolve the glycerine and preservative in water. Heat (a) to 70°C. Add (a) to (b), then stir down to 35°C. Add colour and then perfume.

9 *Sunscreen Lotion (Alcoholic type)*
   Antiviray   10.0
   Isopropyl myristate   40.0
   Toilet spirit   50.0
   Perfume   one or two drops
   Colour (spirit soluble)   one drop

Method: Stir the ingredients together until uniformly mixed.

10 *Sunscreen Lotion (Oily type)*
   Antiviray   10.0
   Isopropyl myristate   40.0
   Mineral oil (cosmetic
     quality)   50.0
   Perfume   one or two drops
   Colour (oil soluble)   one drop
   Preservative (Nipagin M)   one microspatula-full

Method: Dissolve the perfume in the isopropyl myristate. Stir in the antiviray, then the mineral oil. Add the colour and stir well.

11 *Sunscreen/Insect Repellent Cream*
 a Stearic acid   6.0
   Isopropyl myristate   7.0
   Emulsene 1219 (emulsifier)   10.0
   Antiviray   5.0
   Dimethyl phthalate   20.0
 b Triethanolamine   2.0
   Distilled water   50.0
   Preservative (Nipagin M)   one microspatula-full
 c Perfume   one or two drops

Method: Heat (*a*) and (*b*) independently to 75°C and add (*b*) to (*a*) slowly with continuous stirring, adding the perfume when the temperature has fallen to about 35°C.

12 *Sunscreen/Insect Repellent Lotion*
 a Ethylene glycol
     monostearate   2.0
   Emulsene 1220 (emulsifier)   5.0
   Antiviray   10.0
   Dimethyl phthalate   20.0
 b Glycerine   5.0
   Distilled water   58.0
   Preservative (Nipagin M)   one microspatula-full
 c Perfume   one or two drops
 d Colour   one drop

Method: As above, adding colour if required.

13 *Tan and Sunscreen Cream*

Dihydroxyacetone	3.5
Propylene glycol	5.0
Antiviray W.S.	10.0
Toilet spirit	35.0
Distilled water	46.5
Perfume	one or two drops
Preservative (Nipagin M)	one microspatula-full

Method: Dissolve the antiviray and dihydroxyacetone in water. Add the alcohol and propylene glycol. Add the perfume and preservative.

14 Sun Tan Oil

Antiviray	1.0
Liquid paraffin	26.9
Olive oil	40.0
Stearic acid	30.0
Carrot oil	2.0
Fat stabilizer	0.1
Perfume	one or two drops
Preservative (Nipagin M)	one microspatula-full

Method: Dissolve antiviray in the liquid paraffin by heating gently. Add the other substances at room temperature. Perfume, and add the preservative.

15 Sun Tan Oil

Sesame oil	25.0
Mineral oil	50.0
Isopropyl myristate	25.0
Antiviray	one drop
Perfume	one or two drops
Antioxidant (Progallin)	one drop
Preservative (Nipagin M)	one microspatula-full

Method: Mix all the ingredients together.

16 Sun Tan Cream

a	Diglycol stearate "S"	2.0
	Stearic acid	1.5
	Cetyl alcohol	0.5
	Antiviray	5.0
b	Triethanolamine	1.0
	Distilled water	90.0
c	Perfume	one or two drops
	Preservative (Nipagin M)	one microspatula-full

Method: Heat (a) to 75°C. Heat (b) to 75°C. Add (b) to (a). Add (c).

10 SHAVING CREAMS AND LOTIONS

Brushless shaving creams

These are oil in water emulsions and usually consist of mineral oil emulsified in water with a stearic soap. The creams should have the following properties:

1   They must keep the beard moist during the shave.
2   They must lubricate the movement of the razor over the beard.
3   They must spread easily over the face.
4   They must be easily rinsed from the face.
5   The perfume must be correct for the particular emulsion. (See Appendix III).

The creams could contain stearic acid, an alkali such as caustic soda or triethanolamine to neutralize the stearic acid. The oil phase consists of liquid paraffin or white petroleum jelly, lanolin or cetyl alcohol.

Glycerine is the humectant.

Formulae   *Grammes*

1 *a* Stearic acid   20.0
    b Mineral oil   2.0
    c Cetyl alcohol   0.5
    d Potassium hydroxide   1.0
    e Glycerine   7.0
    f Distilled water   69.5
    g Perfume   one or two drops
    h Preservative (Nipagin M) one microspatula-full

Method:
   1 Melt (*a*), (*b*) and (*c*) to 70°C.
   2 Dissolve (*d*) and (*e*) in (*f*), heat to 70°C. Add (1) to (2), stir until cool (35°C). Add the perfume and preservative.

2 *a* Stearic acid   16.0
    b White mineral oil   4.0
    c Lanolin (anhydrous)   3.5
    d Polyethylene glycol 600
        monostearate   3.2
    e Potassium hydroxide   0.8
    f Terpineol   0.3
    g Propylene glycol   4.0
    h Distilled water   68.2
     i Preservative (Nipagin M) one microspatula-full

Method: Melt (*a*), (*b*), (*c*) and (*d*) to 60°C. Dissolve the terpineol in propylene glycol. Heat to 60°C. Dissolve potassium hydroxide in water (heat to 60°C). Stir, add the terpineol dissolved in propylene glycol, then add the mixture of a, b, c and d. Add perfume and preservative.

3 *a*	Isopropyl myristate	2.0
	Stearic acid	25.0
	Acetoglyceride L/C	5.0
b	Triethanolamine	1.0
	Distilled water	56.0
c	Triethanolamine lauryl sulphate	1.0
	Distilled water	10.0
	Preservative (Nipagin M)	one microspatula-full
d	Perfume	one drop

Method: Heat (*a*) and (*b*) independently to 70°C. Add (*b*) to (*a*) with continuous stirring. Add (*c*) to the emulsion at 35°C. Add the perfume.

Shaving soap creams

The functions of a shaving cream are such that:

1 It must produce a rich lather composed of small bubbles because larger ones are too watery.
2 It must not irritate the skin.
3 It must have very good wetting properties.
4 It should be smooth, soft and not lumpy.
5 It must stay on the face and brush, but must be easily removed on rinsing.

These properties will be found in a cream if the correct raw materials are used, such as coconut oil to give a good lather, and the emollient should be either lanolin, glycerine, mineral oil or vaseline.

Formulae *Grammes*

1 *a*	Stearic acid	30.0
	Coconut oil	10.0
	Palm kernel oil	5.0
b	Potassium hydroxide	7.0
	Sodium hydroxide	1.5
	Glycerine	10.0
	Distilled water	36.5
	Preservative (Nipagin M)	one microspatula-full
c	Perfume	one to three drops

Method: Heat (*a*) and (*b*) independently to 75°C. Add (*b*) to (*a*). Stir until emulsion is formed. Add perfume at 35°C.

Note: The preservative and glycerine are dissolved in the water.

Pre-electric shave lotion

The purpose of pre-electric shave lotions is to dry the skin, i.e. to free it from perspiration. The lotion should be astringent and contain oily materials in order to lubricate the hairs and facilitate ease of cutting. Alcohol is the major constituent which dries the skin and causes hair to stand erect. Acetoglyceride L/C gives the emollient effect.

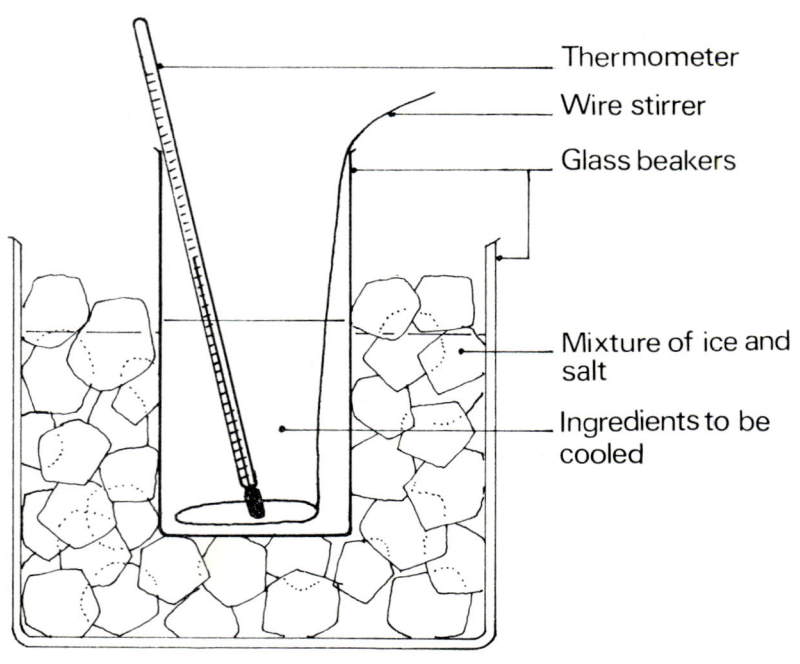

Fig. 10 Diagram to show the method of cooling liquids to temperatures near 0°C. The beaker containing the liquid to be cooled is placed in a large beaker containing a mixture of ice and salt. The liquid should be stirred continuously until the required temperature is reached.

Formulae   *Grammes*

1   Boric acid   2.0
    Menthol (pure)   0.1

Acetoglyceride L/C	12.0
Toilet spirit	85.9
Perfume	three to four drops
Colour (spirit soluble)	one drop

Method: Dissolve all the ingredients in the alcohol in a beaker. Cool to 0°–5°C (see Fig. 10) and filter.

2   a Crodamol ML   15.0
    b Menthol (pure)   0.1
    c Toilet spirit   74.9
    d Perfume   three drops
    e Colour (spirit soluble) one drop

Method: Dissolve (*b*) and (*c*) in (*d*), then add (*a*).

3   Isopropyl myristate   12.0
    Menthol   0.1
    Boric acid   0.5
    Toilet spirit   87.4
    Perfume   three drops
    Colour (spirit soluble)   one drop

Method: Dissolve the menthol and boric acid in half of the spirit. Dissolve the perfume in the remaining spirit. Mix the two solutions together, then add the isopropyl myristate.

After shave lotions

Formulae   *Grammes*

1 a Crodamol DA   1.0
      Polawax   2.0
      Cithrol 10 MS   1.0
      Menthol   0.05
      Cetrimide   0.10
   b Propylene glycol   1.0
      Toilet spirit   12.5
      Carbitol   8.0
      Distilled water   72.85
      Preservative (Nipagin M)   one microspatula-full
      Colour   three drops
   c Di-isopropanolamine (10%
         solution)   1.5
   d Perfume   one drop

Method: Heat (*a*) to 65°–70°C. Heat (*b*) to 70°C over a water bath and add to (*a*), stirring quickly. Heat (*c*) to 60°–65°C, and add to above. Add perfume at 50°C.

2 a Crodamol DA   3.63
   b Toilet spirit   64.20
   c Distilled water   31.90
   d Cetrimide   0.09
   e Menthol or witch hazel   0.18
   f Perfume   three drops
   g Preservative (Nipagin M)   one microspatula-full

Method: Mix (*a*) and (*b*), add (*d*) and (*e*), then add (*c*) and (*g*). Stir. Add perfume and stir. Filter if necessary.

3 a Isopropyl myristate   5.0
   b Toilet spirit   60.0
   c Distilled water   32.4
   d Boric acid   2.4
   e Menthol   0.1
   f Perfume   three drops
   g Colour   one drop
   h Preservative (Nipagin M)   one microspatula-full

Method:

  1 Dissolve (*d*), (*e*) and (*h*) in (*c*).

  2 Mix (*a*) and (*b*). Mix (1) and (2) together. Add (*f*) and (*g*) and stir.

4   Toilet spirit   50.0
      Glycerine   3.0
      Distilled water   47.0
      Perfume   three drops
      Colour   one drop
      Cetrimide   one microspatula-full
      Preservative (Nipagin M)   one microspatula-full

Method: Dissolve the cetrimide and preservative in the water. Add the glycerine and then mix with the alcohol. Colour if necessary, then add the perfume.

5
Other skin cosmetics

1 BATH PREPARATIONS

Bath preparations consist of bath crystals, bath cubes, bath powder and bath oils. They are mainly used for softening the water. The basic materials used are:

Sodium sesquicarbonate ($Na_2CO_3 \cdot NaHCO_2 \cdot 2H_2O$): This substance crystallizes in very fine needle-shaped crystals, sometimes referred to as feather crystals. It is used as a water softener and in bath powders. The crystals are coloured and perfumed to make them more attractive. They are stable, and soluble in water.

Sodium carbonate (Washing soda) ($Na_2CO_3 \cdot 10H_2O$): The crystals are small and resemble peas in shape. The salt contains about 63% of its own weight of water. It dissolves very easily in hot water. If the water is hard, it forms a precipitate of calcium and magnesium carbonates, thus softening the water.

Sodium perborate ($NaBO_3 \cdot 4H_2O$): This can be used to make a bubble-bath by adding about 10% by weight to sodium sesquicarbonate. It has about 10% of available oxygen. The alkali decomposes the perborate in the bath with the evolution of oxygen.

Sodium phosphate ($Na_2HPO_4 \cdot 12H_2O$): This salt is less soluble than sodium carbonate. The solution becomes milky. It effloresces quickly.

Sodium chloride (NaCl) (Common Salt): This salt is composed of colourless cubic crystals. If too much of it is put into a bath of water, it is difficult to obtain a lather. This salt has a refreshing effect on the skin.

Borax ($Na_2B_4O_7 \cdot 10H_2O$): This salt is sometimes blended with those previously mentioned. It has no drying effect on the skin.

Bath powders: These are made from anhydrous sodium carbonate or sesquicarbonate, and borax. The sodium salt of sulphated lauryl alcohol in powder form is sometimes added. This reduces the surface tension and gives added froth.

Colours: The crystals are coloured to give them a more pleasing appearance. The colours most frequently used are yellow, blue, pink, violet and green. Many of the colours can be mixed to give other shades. They can be dissolved in water or in methylated spirit. The amount of colour used depends on the depth of the colour required. The colours can be added in powder form. If this is done, it is advisable to wear rubber gloves for the mixing of the salts and colours.

Perfumes: These could be chosen from verbena, lavender, rose, cologne or pine.

Formulae *Grammes*

1   *Bath Salts*
   a Sodium sesquicarbonate   80.0
   b Borax   20.0
   c Glycerine   one drop
   d Colour   one microspatula-full
   e Perfume   one or two drops

Method: Mix (*a*) and (*b*) together in a mortar. Add (*c*) (in order to hold the colour). Add (*d*) and then add perfume (*e*). Place in a suitable container, e.g. a polythene bag.

2   *Bath Salts*
   a Sodium carbonate (pea
      crystals)   90.0
   b Sodium lauryl sulphate   10.0
   c Glycerine   one drop
   d Colour   one microspatula-full
   e Perfume   one to three drops

Method: As above.

Note: Sodium carbonate is alkaline. Therefore not more than about 50 gms should be used in a bath.

3   *Bubble Bath Salts*
   a Sodium sesquicarbonate
      (feather crystals)   90.0
   b Sodium perborate   10.0
   c Glycerine   one drop
   d Colour   one microspatula-full
   e Perfume   one to three drops

Method: As above.

Note: Only about a handful is needed in a bath.

4   *Softening Powder for the Bath*
     Oatmeal flour   30.0
     Oatmeal bran   10.0
     Ground almonds   10.0
     Wheat flour   10.0

Sodium sesquicarbonate powder	40.0
Perfume	one to three drops
Preservative (Nipagin M)	one microspatula-full

Method: Mix all the ingredients together in a jar.

Note: Use very little in the bath.

5 *Milk Bath*

a	Casein	10.0
	Sodium bicarbonate	80.0
	Sodium carbonate crystals *or* sodium sesquicarbonate crystals	10.0
b	Perfume	one or two drops
	Preservative (Nipagin M)	one microspatula-full

Method: Grind (a) to a fine powder in a mortar and mix well. Add the perfume and preservative.

6 *Foot Bath Salts*

a	Sodium sesquicarbonate (feather crystals)	100.0
b	Glycerine	one drop
c	Colour (green)	one microspatula-full
d	Perfume (Pine)	one or two drops

Method: Mix (a), (b) and (c) together. Add the perfume (d).

7 *Foot Bath Salts*

a	Sodium sulphate (Glauber's salt)	10.0
b	Sodium bicarbonate	70.0
c	Sodium chloride	20.0
d	Perfume	one or two drops

Method: As above.

8 *Foot Bath Salts*

a	Sodium perborate	2.0
b	Sodium bicarbonate	45.0
c	Sodium carbonate crystals	43.0
d	Borax	10.0
e	Perfume	one or two drops

Method: Mix (a), (b), (c) and (d) together in a mortar. Add the perfume (e).

9 *Cream Bath*

Emulsene	5.0
Stearic acid	30.0
Mineral oil	34.9
Wheat germ oil	3.0

Vegetable oil (any type)	27.0
Fat stabilizer	0.1
Preservative (Nipagin M)	one microspatula-full
Perfume	two to three drops

Method: Melt all the ingredients in a beaker. This results in a milky emulsion with the bath water. It lubricates the skin and acts as an emollient.

Bath oils and emulsions

There are two types of bath oils. In one type the perfume is dissolved in the oil, such as mineral oil, and then coloured. In the second type the perfume is dispersed to form a transparent emulsion. It can be coloured and is water soluble.

Formulae *Grammes*

1 Bath Oil

Isopropyl myristate	62.5
Mineral oil (cosmetic quality)	37.5
Colour (if desired)	one microspatula-full
Perfume	three drops
Preservative (Nipagin M)	one microspatula-full

Method: Mix the mineral oil and isopropyl myristate in a beaker. Add colour, perfume and preservative.

2 Bath Oil

Cetyl alcohol *or* Abracol GMS	5.0
Isopropyl myristate	35.0
Mineral oil	30.0
Olive oil	27.0
Carrot oil	3.0
Perfume	one to three drops
Preservative (Nipagin M)	one microspatula-full

Method: Melt all ingredients, with the exception of the perfume in a beaker. Add perfume when the temperature has dropped to 35°C.

3 Bath Oil (*Dispersible*)

Abracol LDS	5.0
Liquid lanolin	10.0
Isopropyl myristate	25.0
Mineral oil *or* vegetable oil	60.0
Perfume or oil of lemon	three drops
Preservative (Nipagin M)	one microspatula-full

Method: As above.

4 *Bath Oil*
   Abracol LDS   5.0
   Mineral oil   80.0
   Oleyl alcohol   15.0
   Perfume   three drops
   Preservative (Nipagin M)   one microspatula-full
   Method: As above.

5 Cithrol No. 6 (Croda)   12.0
   Perfume   one or two drops
   Distilled water   87.0

Method: Dissolve the perfume in the Cithrol. Add the water which has been warmed. Stir slowly.

2 DEODORANTS

Cosmetic preparations intended to reduce body odours function by inhibiting the bacterial decomposition of perspiration. There are two types of sweat glands in the skin (see page 18) and the source of body odour arises from the decomposition of secretion from the apocrine glands.

Aluminium chloride is the active ingredient which is found in most liquid deodorants.

Deodorants

Formulae   *Grammes*

1 *Liquid Deodorant*
   a Aluminium chloride   9.0
   b Aluminium sulphate   4.0
   c Borax   1.0
   d Distilled water   86.0
   e Preservative (Nipagin M) one microspatula-full
   f Perfume   three drops

Method: Measure the water into a large cylinder or beaker. Add preservative. Add (a), (b) and (c) and mix thoroughly. Filter if necessary.

Note: The borax is added in order to liberate traces of boric acid when it reacts with the aluminium chloride. It thus prevents the precipitation of the aluminium hydroxide in the preparation. The aluminium chloride and aluminium sulphate are the active agents which counteract odours.

2 *Solid Cream*
   a Lambutol wax N21
      (emulsifier)   11.5

Beeswax 5.0
Mineral oil 10.0
b Aluminium chloride 5.0
Distilled water 68.5
Preservative (Nipagin M) one microspatula-full
Perfume three drops

Method : Heat the waxes and mineral oil (*a*) to 70°C in a beaker. Heat (*b*) to the same temperature. Add (*b*) to (*a*). Stir until an emulsion is formed. Perfume if required.

3 *Solid Cream*
   a Lambutol N2 (emulsifier) 10.0
     Paraffin wax 10.0
     Olive oil 5.0
   b Aluminium chloride 15.0
     Glycerine 5.0
     Distilled water 55.0
     Preservative (Nipagin M) one microspatula-full
   c Perfume three drops

Method : Melt (*a*) in a beaker to 70°C. Heat (*b*) to 70°C. Add (*b*) to (*a*) and stir until emulsified. Add the perfume at 35°C.

4 *Cream*
   a Sunflower oil 7.5
   b Lambutol wax 2.5
   c Beeswax 1.0
   d Glycerine 5.0
   e Aluminium chloride 15.0
   f Distilled water 69.0
   g Preservative (Nipagin M) one microspatula-full
   h Perfume three drops

Method : Melt (*a*), (*b*) and (*c*) to 75°C. Mix (*d*), (*e*) and (*g*) and 40 parts of water and heat until dissolved. Adjust the temperature to 75°C. Add to the molten oil phase. Stir until emulsion is cold, then add the remaining water.

5 *Lotion*
   a Aluminium chloride 9.0
   b Aluminium sulphate 14.0
   c Borax 1.0
   d Distilled water 76.0
   e Preservative (Nipagin M) one microspatula-full
   f Perfume three drops

Method : Mix (*a*), (*b*) and (*c*) together. Add the water, and preservative, mix thoroughly.

Antiperspirants

1 *Cream*
   - a Petroleum jelly — 2.5
     Cetyl alcohol — 2.5
     Paraffin wax — 5.0
     Mineral oil — 5.0
     Emulsifier (Abracol LDS) — 5.0
   - b Distilled water — 35.0
     Glycerine — 5.0
   - c Aluminium chloride — 40.0
   - d Perfume — three drops
     Preservative (Nipagin M) — one microspatula-full

Method: Heat (a) to 75°C. Heat (b) to 75°C. Add (b) to (a). Add (c) when the temperature falls to 35°C. Add the perfume and preservative.

2 *Cream*
   - a Mineral oil — 7.5
     Petroleum jelly — 2.5
     Spermaceti — 5.0
     Emulsifier (Abracol LDS) — 15.0
   - b Glycerine — 5.0
     Distilled water — 25.0
   - c Aluminium chloride — 40.0
   - d Perfume — three drops
     Preservative (Nipagin M) — one microspatula-full

Method: As above.

3 *Cream*
   - a Mineral oil — 7.5
     Petroleum jelly — 5.0
     Abracol LDS — 3.5
     Abracol GSP — 15.0
   - b Glycerine — 5.0
     Distilled water — 24.0
   - c Aluminium chloride — 40.0
   - d Perfume — three drops
     Preservative (Nipagin M) — one microspatula-full

Method: As above.

4 *Cream*
   - a Glyceryl monostearate — 17.0
   - b Spermaceti — 9.0
   - c Glycerine — 3.9
   - d Distilled water — 37.0
   - e Preservative (Nipagin M) — 1.0

f	Aluminium sulphate	15.0
g	Distilled water	15.0
h	Titanium dioxide	2.0
i	Phenoxetol	1.0
j	Perfume	three drops

Method: Dissolve (f) in (g), then add (i) and stir in (h). Heat (c), (d) and (e) in a beaker to 90°C. Heat (a) and (b) to 90°C. Add to the water phase with constant stirring until an emulsion is formed. When cool, add the mixture of (f), (g) and (h).

Note: Titanium dioxide serves as a filler to give the cream more body.

5   Lotion

Glycerine	2.0
Cetrimide	0.5
Propylene glycol	5.0
Distilled water	12.5
Aluminium chloride	30.0
Toilet spirit	50.0
Perfume	three drops
Preservative (Nipagin M)	one microspatula-full

Method: Dissolve the cetrimide in the propylene glycol with gentle heat (40°C) over a water bath. Allow to cool. Mix the remainder of the materials together. Add the cetrimide solution.

6   Lotion

Propylene glycol	2.5
Toilet spirit	45.0
Aluminium chloride	10.0
Distilled water	42.5
Perfume	three drops
Preservative (Nipagin M)	one microspatula-full

Method: Dissolve the perfume in the toilet spirit. Add the propylene glycol. Dissolve the aluminium chloride and preservative in the water and add this to the toilet spirit and propylene glycol. Stir thoroughly.

3 FACE AND TALCUM POWDERS

Face powders are classified according to bulk density. They should impart a smooth velvet-like finish to the skin by hiding any shine due to the secretions of the sebaceous and sweat glands. Also the powders must not have a clown-like appearance—that is, too white and heavy. They must have reasonably lasting properties and have a pleasing odour. The colours of the powders should match the colouring of the skin.

In order to impart all these properties, the raw materials used are:

1   *For covering*, that is to cover skin defects (e.g. enlarged pores, etc.)—titanium dioxide, zinc oxide, kaolin or magnesium oxide.
2   *For slip*, i.e. to help the spreading of the powder and to give the skin a smooth feeling—talc, zinc stearate, starch, lithium stearate or satinex.
3   *For absorbing* the sebaceous secretions and perspiration, thus reducing the shine—either precipitated chalk, magnesium carbonate, starch or kaolin.
4   *To make the powder adhere* to the skin—the metallic soaps such as the magnesium and zinc salts of the various fatty acids.
5   *To give the necessary bloom* (the smooth, velvet-like appearance) to the skin—chalk or starch.

Most of the raw materials can be found in the laboratory of any school. There are, however, a few exceptions. The basic main material in face powder is *talc*. This is an abundant mineral found in many parts of the world. It is a hydrated magnesium silicate. Any impurities present in the mineral can influence the physical characteristics of the powdered material a great deal. If the calcium content is high and present in the talc as calcium silicate, the powder will be abrasive. It is better to select a talc with a low calcium content. Other impurities in the talc are iron compounds such as iron(III) oxide or magnesium iron(III) silicate. These tend to give the talc a greyish colour and render it useless for cosmetic formulation. Talc is mined in France, Italy, U.S.A., India, Egypt and China.

Starch is found in roots, rhizomes, fruits and in the seeds of most plants. It is also obtained from potatoes, rice, wheat and corn starch. Maize starch is used to a limited degree in powders now.

Magnesium Carbonate (light): This is a white powder which can absorb liquids well. It is often used to incorporate the perfume for use in the final mixing of a face or talcum powder.

Kaolin (China Clay): This is a naturally occurring mineral found in Cornwall, and in Georgia and South Carolina in the U.S.A. The kaolins are hydrated aluminium silicates, white to pale cream in colour, and can be used to help powders cling.

Zinc Oxide is a white powder which is used to soothe the skin. It is used to give opacity to the powder.

Calcium Carbonate: This imparts a greater density to the powder. It is produced from minerals such as limestone, marble, chalk, etc. The crude ore is crushed, washed and ground to give different grades of particle sizes.

Lithium Stearate is a fluffy material of low density. It is particularly suitable for baby powder.

Boric Acid is used in some powders for its antiseptic properties.

Satinex is a fine white powder. It has a good colour and is better than magnesium stearate and zinc stearate as:

   1 It has a softer texture and is lighter to touch.

   2 It has a lower density than either magnesium or zinc stearate.

   3 It has a much better covering power than the usual stearates, without increasing "whiteness". Face powders incorporating satinex often require less pigment. It can also be added to lipstick formulations (2.0–3.0%). The addition of satinex gives a creaming effect and produces a lipstick with a smooth film. Satinex should be mixed with the eosin and colours.

Colours. The colours that are used for face powders must be bright and still give an appearance of being delicate and alive. They must be selected with great care. Popular colours are cream, rachel, brunette.

Pigments: Brown, yellow and the red oxides of iron; others such as cobalt, green, ultramarine and blue.

Lakes: Carmines and some of the dyestuffs.

To obtain colours for the powders, it is necessary to mix certain of the various pigments and dyes, for example:

Cream or Rachel—yellow ochre or cadmium sulphide.

Brunette—burnt sienna and traces of eosin solution.

Naturelle—pink lakes blended with yellow ochres and a little burnt sienna.

Peach—pink lakes blended with orange lakes or dyestuffs.

Other colours can, of course, be made by experimenting with different shades.

Perfumes. The quantity of perfume used normally varies according to individual requirement. The perfume must be added to a small quantity of one of the absorbent powders composing the base. The type of perfume will vary with individual preference, but the following are some suggestions which can be obtained from the sources listed in Appendix III:

Face Powders—amber, chypre, bouquet.

Talcum powders—eau de Cologne, lavender, bouquet, fougere.

Face Powders

Formulae *Grammes*

1.
Satinex	12.0
Zinc oxide	10.0
Calcium carbonate	20.0
Titanium dioxide	5.0
Talc	53.0
Colouring	five to ten microspatula-full
Perfume	five drops

Method: Add the perfume (by means of a dropper) to part of the calcium or magnesium carbonate and allow to stand for some time. Mix the pigments with a proportion of the talc. Add the remaining powders and the perfume mixture. Mix and sieve, either by means of a silk mesh or an old washed nylon stocking.

2. *Powder with Reduced Covering Power*

Satinex	12.0
Zinc oxide	10.0
Calcium carbonate (light)	25.0
Talc	53.0
Colouring	one microspatula-full
Perfume	five drops

Method: As above.

3.
Zinc stearate	5.0
Zinc oxide	10.0
Calcium carbonate (light)	20.0
Talc	58.0
Titanium dioxide	2.0
Magnesium carbonate (light)	5.0
Colouring	one microspatula-full
Perfume	five drops

Method: As above.

4. *Light Powder*

Talc	64.0
Kaolin	20.0
Calcium carbonate (light)	5.0
Zinc oxide	5.0
Zinc stearate	5.0
Magnesium carbonate	1.0
Colouring	five to ten microspatula-full
Perfume	five drops

Method: As above.

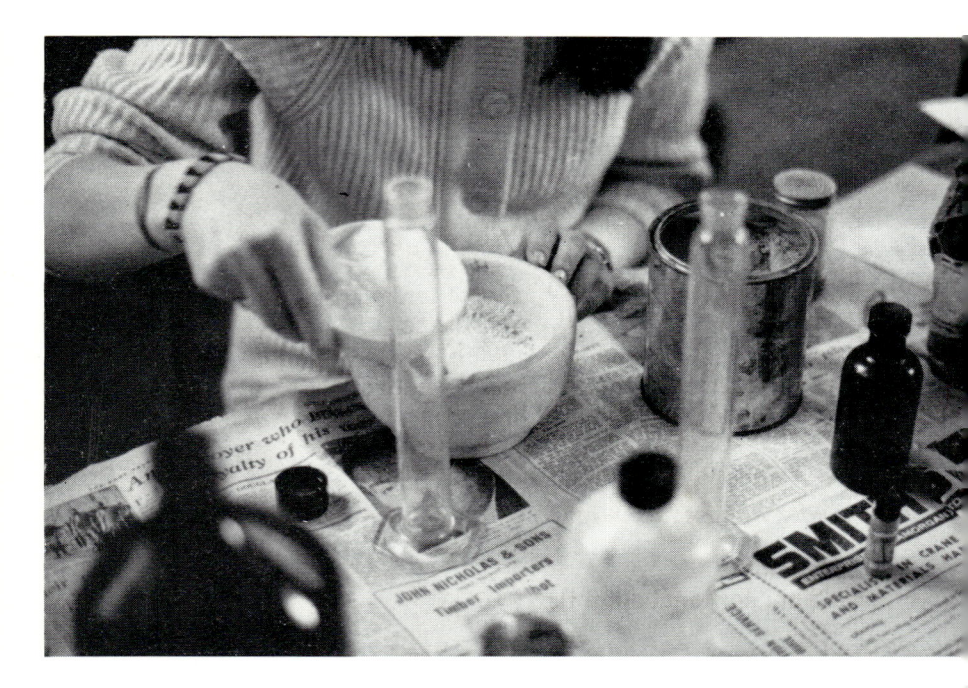

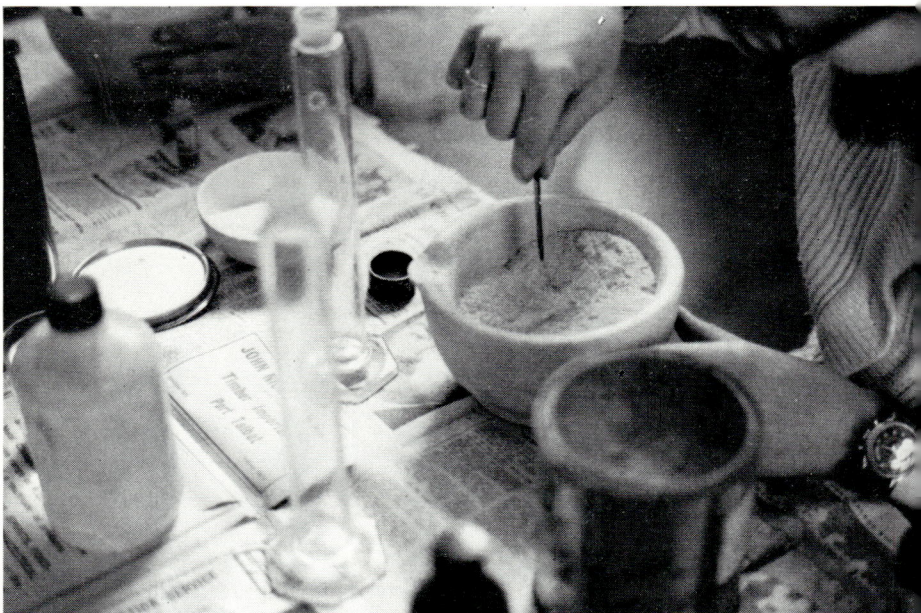

Fig. 11 Mixing face powders.

5 *Medium Powder*
Talc	40.0
Kaolin	40.0
Calcium carbonate (light)	5.0
Zinc oxide	7.0
Zinc stearate	7.0
Magnesium carbonate	1.0
Colouring	one microspatula-full
Perfume	five drops

Method: As above.

Talcum powders

These are used to absorb perspiration and to prevent chafing. Talcum powders consist mainly of talc, with small proportions of a metallic stearate and precipitated calcium carbonate (chalk) or magnesium carbonate (light). Boric acid is sometimes used for its antiseptic action. The proportion of metallic stearate used in talcum powders is from 4–10%.

Formulae   *Grammes*

1 | | |
   |---|---|
   | Satinex | 7.0 |
   | Talc | 88.0 |
   | Magnesium carbonate (light) | 5.0 |
   | Perfume | five drops |
   | Preservative (Nipagin M) | one microspatula-full |

Method: Add the perfume to part of the calcium or magnesium carbonate and allow to stand for some time. Add the remaining powders and the perfume mixture. Mix and sieve (as in the recipe for face powder).

2 | | |
   |---|---|
   | Zinc stearate | 5.0 |
   | Calcium carbonate (light) | 25.0 |
   | Talc | 70.0 |
   | Perfume | five drops |
   | Preservative (Nipagin M) | one microspatula-full |

Method: As above.

3 *Baby Powder*
Magnesium stearate	5.0
Magnesium carbonate (light)	5.0
Talc	87.5
Boric acid	2.5
Perfume	five drops
Preservative (Nipagin M)	one microspatula-full

Method: As above.

4   *Baby Powder*
Talc	70.0
Kaolin	20.0
Magnesium stearate	4.0
Boric acid	3.0
Satinex	3.0
Perfume (if required)	one drop
Preservative (Nipagin M)	one microspatula-full

Method: As above.

5   *Baby Powder*
Talc	84.0
Kaolin	10.0
Boric acid	4.0
Satinex	2.0
Perfume (if required)	one drop
Preservative (Nipagin M)	one microspatula-full

Method: As above.

6   *Medicated Dusting Powder*
Sodium propanedioate	20.0
Talc	80.0
Preservative (Nipagin M)	one microspatula-full

Method: Mix all ingredients together in a mortar, and sieve.

7   *Foot Powder*
Boric acid	10.0
Starch or kaolin	45.0
Talc	45.0
Menthol	one drop

Method: As above.

8   *Foot Powder*
Boric acid	11.0
Starch	20.0
Talc	69.0
Preservative (Nipagin M)	one microspatula-full

Method: As above.

4 EYE COSMETICS

Formulae   *Grammes*

1   *Eye Shadow*
    a | | |
       |---|---|
       | Castor oil | 45.0 |
       | Acetoglyceride L/C | 10.0 |
       | Isopropyl myristate | 2.0 |

b	Lanolin	3.0
	Mineral oil	2.0
	Acetoglyceride S/C/2	5.0
	Beeswax	7.0
	Ozokerite	5.0
	Carnauba wax	2.0
	Candelilla wax	7.0
c	Colours	10.0
	Titanium dioxide	2.0
	Preservative (Nipagin M)	one microspatula-full
d	Perfume	one drop

Method: Part (a)—blend all ingredients together. Stir in part (c). Part (b)—melt waxes to 78°–80°C Heat the mixed oils and colours to the same temperature and mix into the melted waxes. Stir, add the perfume, mix and pour into a mould. If preferred, the titanium dioxide may be added at the same stage as the perfume.

Note: Small quantities can be made in different shades by taking portions of (a) and (b) and adding different colours to each. 50 g of eye shadow base suffices for two pupils.

2   *Eye Shadow*

Liquid lanolin	4.0
Beeswax	4.0
Microcrystalline wax	8.0
Isopropyl myristate	36.0
Petroleum jelly	48.0
Preservative (Nipagin M)	one microspatula-full
Perfume	one drop
Colour	one to ten microspatula-full

Method: Melt all the ingredients, with the exception of perfume and colour, together in a beaker. When cool (35°C), add perfume. Take a small amount of base and add colour. If a paler colour is required, add titanium dioxide.

3   *Eye Shadow*

a	Isopropyl myristate	32.0
	Petroleum jelly	17.0
b	Paraffin wax	16.0
	Cetyl alcohol	2.0
c	Zinc oxide	18.0
	Colour	15.0
	Preservative (Nipagin M)	one microspatula-full
d	Perfume	one drop

Method: Melt together the isopropyl myristate and petroleum jelly (a). Stir in part (c). When thoroughly mixed, melt the waxes (b) and add to the oil paste. Stir well. Add the perfume, then mould.

4   Eye Shadow

Base
- Petroleum jelly   23.0
- Beeswax   24.0
- Spermaceti   3.0
- Mineral oil   50.0
- Preservative (Nipagin M)   one microspatula-full

Colours   one microspatula-full

Method: Melt together all ingredients with the exception of the colours. Allow to cool. Divide the base into separate portions. Add the required colours to these portions. Re-melt and pour into containers.

5   Powder Eye Shadow

a
- Calcium carbonate   5.0
- Satinex   one microspatula-full
- Talc   25.0
- Magnesium stearate   50.0

b
- Titanium dioxide   10.0
- Colours   10.0
- Preservative (Nipagin M)   one microspatula-full

Method: Mix (b) together and sieve through a clean nylon stocking or fine muslin. Add (a) to (b) and mix thoroughly until uniform. Place in eye shadow case.

Note: Smaller quantities can be made by taking about 25 g of the base and adding colour as required.

6   Eye Liner

a
- Emulsene 1220 (Abrac)   1.25
- Distilled water   39.75

b
- Glycerine   3.25
- Alcohol   24.0
- Colour (Anstead brown, or any colour preferred)   31.75
- Preservative (Nipagin M01 or Nipasol M001)   one microspatula-full

Method:

(a)   Prepare a dispersion of Emulsene 1220 in water.

(b)   Dissolve the preservative in the glycerine with the aid of gentle heat and disperse the colour in this mixture. Remove the mixture from the heat, add the alcohol and mix with stirring. Add (b) to (a) and stir well.

Note: It may be found that the viscosity of the colour varies slightly so that the weight given above may also vary. Should this be the case, the quantity of water used in the preparation of part (*a*) can be suitably adjusted to give the desired consistency to the finished product.

Mascara

This should be capable of being applied evenly without causing the eyelashes to stick together. It should dry quickly and be reasonably permanent, non-irritant and non-toxic. It can be formulated in cream, liquid or cake form.

Lake Mascara: This is produced from a soap, usually triethanolamine stearate, modified with oils, waxes and colours.

Liquid Mascara may be prepared from an alcoholic solution or resin in which carbon black is suspended. A small amount of castor oil could be introduced into the formula.

Cream Mascara can be produced by milling a pigment into a cream type base.

Formulae   *Grammes*

1   *Mascara*
  a Carnauba wax   5.0
     Beeswax   15.0
     Isopropyl myristate   3.0
     Stearic acid   35.0
     Abracol S.L.G.   5.0
  b Triethanolamine   15.0
  c Sodium alginate   7.0
     Ultramarine blue   12.0
     Carbon black   2.0
     Titanium dioxide   1.0
     Perfume   one drop
     Preservative (Nipagin M) one microspatula-full

Method: Melt part (*a*) at 85°C and to it add part (*b*) heated to 80°C. Stir. Remove from the heat and while still molten, add part (*c*) with stirring and continue stirring until smooth. Re-melt and mould.

2   *Cream Mascara*
     Beeswax   4.0
     Spermaceti   4.0
     Cetyl alcohol   2.0
     Cocoa butter   6.0

Petroleum jelly	64.0
Colour, plus Titanium dioxide	20.0
Preservative (Nipagin M)	one microspatula-full
Perfume	one drop

Method: Melt the ingredients together. Add preservative and colour.

3   Block Mascara

Glyceryl monostearate	60.0
Paraffin wax	15.0
Carnauba wax	7.0
Lanolin	8.0
Carbon black	10.0
Preservative (Nipagin M)	one microspatula-full

Method: Melt all the ingredients together. Add preservative and colour. Pour into moulds or cases.

4   Block Mascara

a	Isopropyl myristate	12.0
	Abracol GMS	30.0
	Stearic acid	20.0
	Beeswax	11.0
b	Triethanolamine	2.0
	Distilled water	20.0
c	Colours	5.0
	Perfume	one drop
	Preservative (Nipagin M)	one microspatula-full

Method: Heat part (*a*) to 85°C with constant stirring. Heat part (*b*) to 85°C. Add (*b*) to (*a*). Mix thoroughly and form an emulsion. Allow to cool, stirring meanwhile. Add (*c*). Re-melt. Pour into moulds.

5 LIPSTICKS

Formulae   *Grammes*

1

Castor oil	60.0
Lanolin, anhydrous	12.0
Candellila wax	9.0
Isopropyl myristate	8.0
White beeswax	5.0
Carnauba wax	3.0
Ozokerite	3.0
Flavour (usually rose)	one drop
Eosin	one microspatula-full
Colours	one to fifteen microspatula-full

OTHER SKIN COSMETICS 83

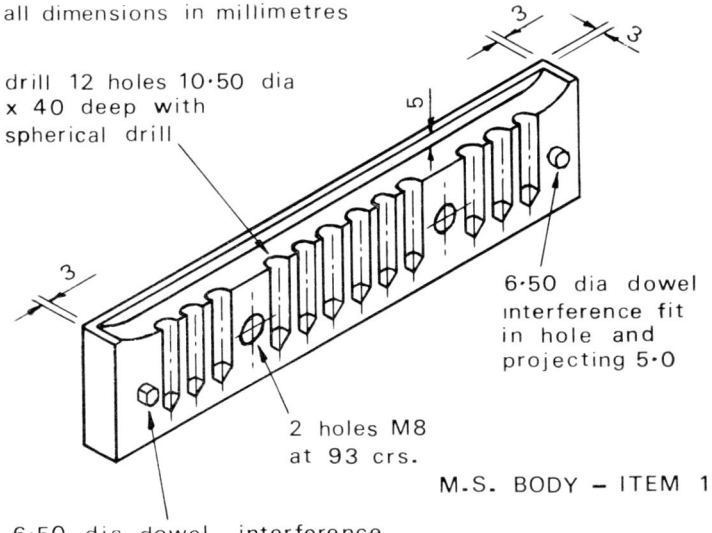

all dimensions in millimetres

drill 12 holes 10·50 dia x 40 deep with spherical drill

6·50 dia dowel interference fit in hole and projecting 5·0

2 holes M8 at 93 crs.

M.S. BODY – ITEM 1

6·50 dia dowel interference fit in hole with two flats to facilitate assembly

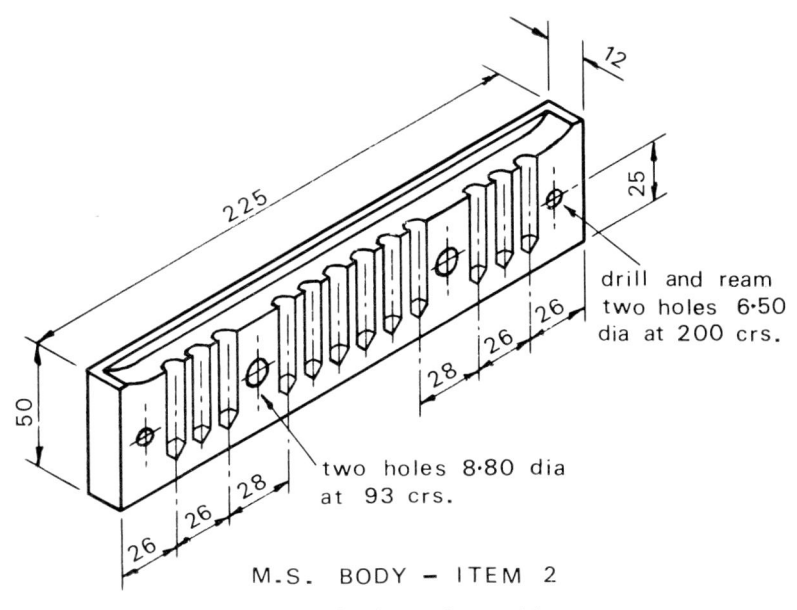

drill and ream two holes 6·50 dia at 200 crs.

two holes 8·80 dia at 93 crs.

M.S. BODY – ITEM 2

Fig. 12   Diagram of a lipstick mould.

24
10
18

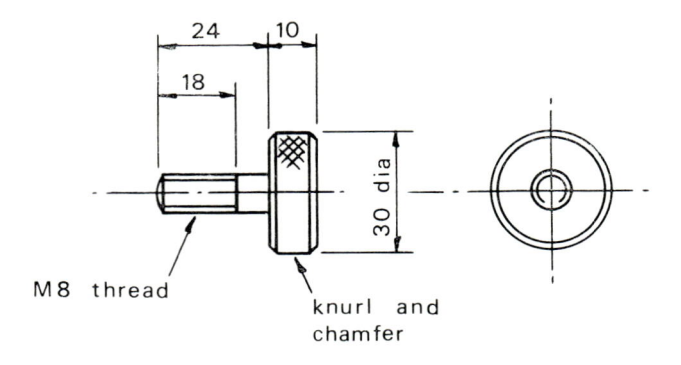

M8 thread

knurl and chamfer

30 dia

MILD STEEL BOLTS – ITEM 3

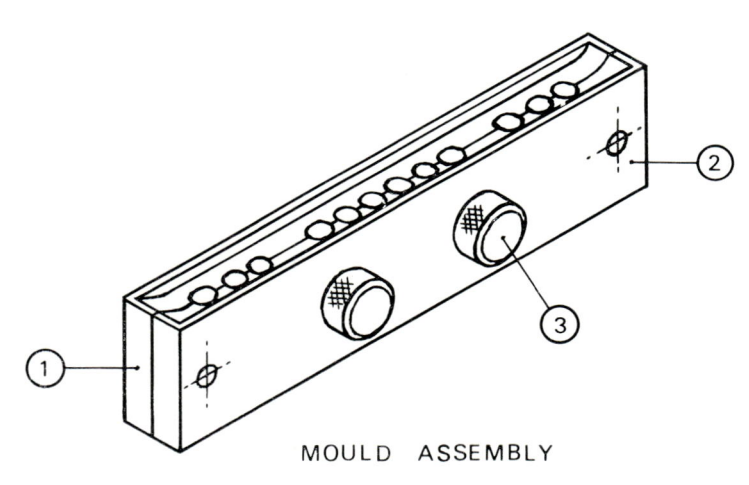

MOULD ASSEMBLY

all parts to be machined to a smooth finish and chromium plated

Fig. 12   Diagram of a lipstick mould.

Perfume		one drop
Preservative (Nipagin M)		one microspatula-full
or (0.25 g Nipasol M		
+ 0.02 g Progallin)		

Method: Weigh the ingredients very carefully. Then take a clean beaker and melt all the oils and waxes together with eosin and preservative. Add perfume and flavouring. This base is sufficient for making about 18–24 lipsticks. If more than one colour is desired, about ¼ of the base is taken and mixed together with the required colour. This is then melted down and poured into a mould and allowed to set. Each stick is then removed and passed through a bunsen flame quickly to give gloss. If muted colours are required, the colours are mixed with titanium dioxide to the required shade.

Note: The eosin in the lipstick can be left out if anyone is allergic to this.

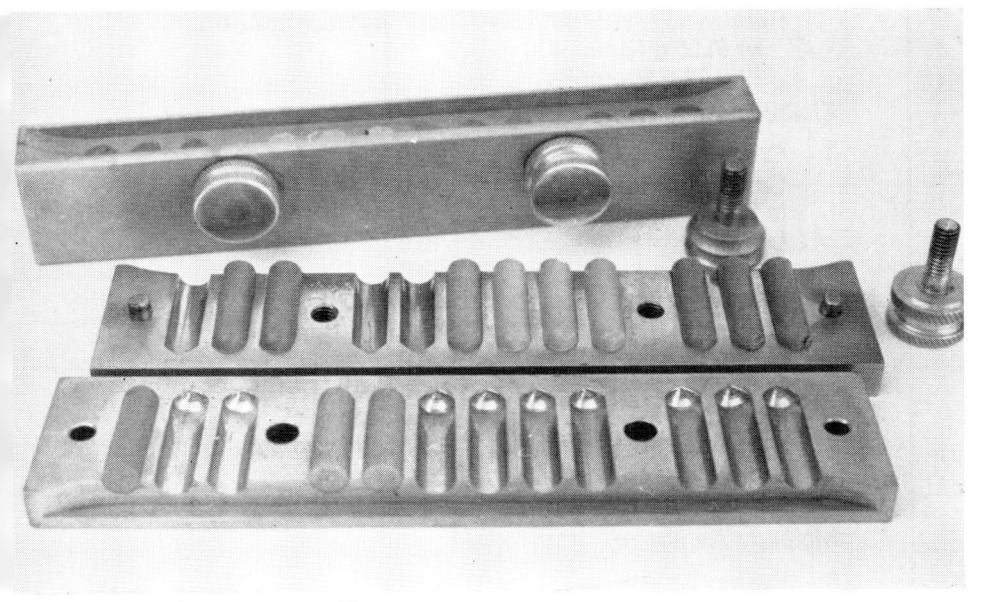

Fig. 13 A lipstick mould.

2	White beeswax	17.0
	Ceresine wax	33.5
	Lanolin	5.5
	White petroleum jelly	27.0
	Cetyl alcohol	6.0
	Olive oil	11.0
	Eosin	one microspatula-full

	Colours	one microspatula-full
	Flavour	one drop
	Perfume	one drop
	Preservative (Nipagin M) or (0.25 g Nipasol M + 0.02 g Progallin)	one microspatula-full

Method: As above.

3	White beeswax	36.0
	Lanolin	8.0
	White petroleum jelly	36.0
	Cetyl alcohol	6.0
	Castor oil	8.0
	Carnauba wax	5.0
	Colours	one to fifteen microspatula-full
	Flavour	one drop
	Perfume	one drop
	Preservative (Nipagin M) or (0.25 g Nipasol M + 0.02 g Progallin)	one microspatula-full

Method: As above.

4	Castor oil	60.0
	Candellila wax	8.0
	Isopropyl myristate	7.5
	Lanolin	10.0
	Beeswax	4.5
	Carnauba wax	2.5
	Ozokerite	2.5
	Colours	5.0
	Flavour	one drop
	Perfume	one drop
	Preservative (Nipagin M) or (0.25 g Nipasol M + 0.02 g Progallin)	one microspatula-full

Method: As above.

5	Carnauba wax	16.0
	Ozokerite	16.0
	Lanolin	24.0
	Liquid paraffin	24.0
	Propylene glycol (eosin solvent)	10.0
	Eosin	7.5
	Titanium dioxide	1.0
	Colours	one to fifteen microspatula-full
	Flavour	1.5

	Perfume	one drop
	Preservative (Nipagin M)	one microspatula-full
	or (0.25 g Nipasol M	
	+ 0.02 g Progallin)	

Method : As above.

6	Castor oil	60.0
	Lanolin	12.0
	Candellila wax	9.0
	Isopropyl myristate	8.0
	Beeswax	5.0
	Carnauba wax	3.0
	Ozokerite	3.0
	Eosin	3.0
	Colours	fifteen microspatula-full
	Flavour	one drop
	Perfume	one drop
	Preservative (Nipagin M)	one microspatula-full
	or (0.25 g Nipasol M	
	+ 0.02 g Progallin)	

Method : As above.

7	Castor oil	60.0
	Lanolin	5.0
	Candellila wax	7.0
	Beeswax	7.0
	Carnauba wax	3.0
	Ozokerite	3.0
	Fluorescein	3.0
	Colours	2.0
	Flavour	one drop
	Perfume	two drops
	Preservative (Nipagin M)	one microspatula-full
	or (0.25 g Nipasol M	
	+ 0.02 g Progallin)	

Method : As above.

8	Carnauba wax	16.0
	Ozokerite	20.0
	Liquid paraffin	24.0
	Peanut or soya oil	20.0
	Oleyl alcohol	10.0
	Eosin and colours	9.0
	Titanium dioxide	1.0
	Flavour	one drop
	Perfume	one drop
	Preservative (Nipagin M)	one microspatula-full
	or (0.25 g Nipasol M	
	+ 0.02 g Progallin)	

Method : As above.

Note: If more than one shade of colour is required, weigh a quarter of the base (i.e. 22.5 g) and mix this with 2.5 g of eosin, colour and titanium dioxide.

9 a *Oil Mixture*

Castor oil	44.0
Acetoglyceride L/C	7.0
Acetoglyceride S/C	2.5
Lanolin	2.0
Isopropyl myristate	2.0

b *Eosin Mixture*

Propylene glycol monomyristate	12.0
Propylene glycol	3.0
Eosin	2.0–3.0

c *Wax Mixture*

Beeswax	7.5
Candellila wax	7.0
Ozokerite wax	5.0
Carnauba wax	5.0
d Colours	5.0
e Perfume	one drop
Preservative (Nipagin M) or (0.25 g Nipasol M + 0.02 g Progallin)	

Method: Melt together the oil constituents (75°C). Add the colours and mix. Make a solution of part (*b*) by mixing the ingredients together, then stir into part (*a*). Add the melted wax constituents and stir until evenly dispersed. Add the perfume and preservative and re-stir. Re-melt and pour into a mould. Finally, allow the mixture to set, and then remove each stick and pass it through bunsen flame to give gloss.

10

Novol (cosmetic grade oleyl alcohol)	20.0
Castor oil	40.0
Candellila wax	10.0
Carnauba wax	10.0
Volpo No. 3 (solvent)	20.0
Flavour	one drop
Colours	fifteen microspatula-full
Perfume	one drop
Preservative (Nipagin M) or (0.25 g Nipasol M + 0.02 g Progallin)	one microspatula-full

Method: Dissolve eosin in the Volpo No. 3 with heating. Add the Novol to this solution, then add the oil phase after heating to 70°C. Add the colours, mix thoroughly, then add the remaining ingredients. Mix thoroughly, then pour into moulds.

6 BEAUTY MASKS

The use of beauty masks dates back to the time of Pharaoh's Egypt, but no accounts have been given of the actual ingredients used. According to legend, Nero's wife used a mixture of which the milk was provided by the famous drove of asses. This is the first known example of casein, the protein of milk, being used for a mask. This formula was re-discovered in Henry III's time. Today, beauty masks and packs are as popular as ever. They help to produce a sense of warmth and tightening of the skin.

A mask is usually a smooth paste, and after application to the skin it should very quickly form a coating which can be easily peeled off when required. The mask absorbs the grease and the dirt from the skin by the action of the colloidal and absorptive earths and clays. When the mask is finally removed from the skin, the surface skin dirt is removed with it.

The effects of the masks can be stimulating, refreshing, softening, cleansing and astringent. Some masks can induce perspiration.

Properties of face masks

1   They should be smooth and free from gritty particles and unpleasant odours. In powder form, they should be easily dispersed in water to produce a good paste.
2   They should be easily removed from the face after use without causing pain or discomfort.
3   They must be harmless to the skin and non-toxic.
4   They should be quick-drying on the face.
5   Any residual matter left should be easily removed by water.

Types of masks

1   Astringent masks: These are the masks based on clays and earths and are the most widely used. The basic materials used are kaolin, china clay, fuller's earth and other materials such as skin softening agents, bleaching agents and astringents (which close the pores)—strong astringents such as lactic acid, potassium and aluminium sulphates or weak astringents such as chalk, witch hazel, orange flower water, fruit juices, etc.

2   Wax masks: These consist of paraffin wax of a suitable melting point, or of mixtures of waxes with petroleum jelly or cetyl alcohol. These masks are melted and brushed on hot

(35°–40°C). They will produce a great deal of perspiration and, in doing so, help to remove dirt and impurities from the skin surface.

3 Albuminous and casein masks: These contain the milk protein casein, glycerine, powdered borax or albumen, lecithin, egg, etc., water and preservative. They have a cleansing and softening effect on the skin.

4 Gelatine masks: These are solid gels composed of glycerine, gelatine and gum tragacanth. Zinc oxide, camphor, kaolin, honey, titanium dioxide, etc. can be added. These masks cause a tightening of the skin and are cleansing and softening.

Formulae   *Grammes*

1 *Gelatine Mask*
   Gum tragacanth   2.2
   Glycerine   2.5
   Gelatine   2.3
   Honey   4.5
   Distilled water   86.0
   Zinc oxide   2.5
   Preservative (Nipagin M
     or Nipasol M)   one microspatula-full

Method: Mix the glycerine with the gum tragacanth. Add the gelatine and water and raise the temperature. Any solids should be mixed in the hot solution, first moistening the solids with glycerine so that they will disperse more easily. These masks must be heated first and then applied to the skin whilst hot (35°C).

2 *Casein Mask*
   Casein   20.0
   Glycerine   5.0
   Distilled water   75.0
   Borax   one microspatula-full
   Preservative (Nipagin M   one microspatula-full
     or Nipasol M)

Method: Moisten the casein with the glycerine. Dissolve this in the water together with the preservative and borax (which has previously been heated to 60°C).

3 *Face Mask for Greasy Skin*
   Kaolin   80.0
   Triethanolamine   3.0
   Magnesium carbonate   12.0
   Starch (rice)   5.0

Tragacanth powder　　　one microspatula-full

Method: Mix the tragacanth with the triethanolamine in a mortar, then mix in the kaolin, magnesium carbonate and rice starch.

4　*Face Mask for Dry Skin*
　　Starch　　　　　　　　　　20.0
　　Kaolin　　　　　　　　　　20.0
　　Cold cream　　　　　　　　20.0
　　Cetyl alcohol　　　　　　　2.0
　　Wheat germ oil　　　　　　5.0
　　Distilled water with borax　33.0

Method: Add the Borax to the distilled water and heat to 75°C. Mix the starch and kaolin together. Then mix all the ingredients to form a paste. Allow the temperature to drop to 35°C before applying the mask to the face.

5　*Fuller's Earth Mask*
　　Fuller's earth　　　　　　　40.0
　　Glycerine　　　　　　　　　2.0
　　Sodium perborate　　　　　10.0
　　Starch paste　　　　　　　　40.0
　　Tincture of benzoin　　　　7.0
　　Petitgrain oil　　　　　　　1.0

Method: Moisten the Fuller's earth with glycerine. Add the sodium perborate and benzoin and oil. Then mix this with the starch paste in a mortar.

6　*Mask Toner*
　　Colloidal kaolin*　　　　　　90.0
　　Tomato juice　　　　　　　　8.0
　　Witch hazel　　　　　　　　2.0
　　Perfume　　　　　　　　　　one to three drops
　　Preservative (Nipagin M)　　one microspatula-full

Method: Add the witch hazel to the colloidal kaolin, stir in the tomato juice, add the preservative and perfume.

7　*A second type* can be made by adding other juices:
　　Colloidal kaolin*　　　　　　85.0
　　Strawberry juice　　　　　　10.0
　　Lemon juice　　　　　　　　5.0
　　Witch hazel　　　　　　　　one drop
　　Perfume　　　　　　　　　　one drop
　　Preservative (Nipagin M)　　one microspatula-full

Method: As above.

　*　Colloidal kaolin is made by adding 8 g distilled water, a small portion at a time, to 10 g kaolin powder and mixing thoroughly.

8   *Yeast Mask*

Wheat germ oil	90.0
Baker's yeast	10.0
Perfume	one drop
Preservative (Nipagin M)	one microspatula-full

Method: Dissolve the yeast in the wheat germ oil. Add the preservative and perfume.

9   *Cream Mask for Greasy Skin*

a	Spermaceti	5.0
	Stearin	5.0
	Vegetable oil	9.0
	Vitamin F	2.0
	Emulsene 1219	4.0
	Preservative (Nipagin M)	one microspatula-full
b	Sorbitol	5.0
	(moistener, conditioner)	
	Manucol	68.0
	Aqueous solution	2.0
c	Biosulphur powder	one microspatula-full

Method: Melt (a) to 65°C. Heat (b) to 65°C and add (c) to this. Add (b) to (a). Stir the cream until the temperature drops to 35°C.

10   *Moisturizing Cream Mask*

a	Emulsene	4.0
	Spermaceti	5.0
	Stearin	5.0
	Vegetable oil	8.0
	Carrot oil	4.0
	Preservative (Nipagin M)	one microspatula-full
b	Sorbitol solution	5.0
	Sodium alginate	64.0
	Hygroplex HHG	5.0
c	Perfume	one to three drops

Method: Melt (a) to 65°C. Heat (b) to 65°C. Stir (b) into (a). Cool to 35°C. Add the perfume and homogenize.

6
Hair, nails and teeth

1 STRUCTURE AND GROWTH OF HAIR

A hair is composed of a shaft and a root. The shaft extends outwards from the skin surface, and consists of a cuticle, a cortex of keratinized epidermal cells, which contain the pigment, and a medulla or central canal. The root is encased in a follicle and is found deep in the dermis of the skin (see Fig. 5). It expands, at the lower end, into a bulb which rests upon the papilla. Through the papilla run the blood vessels which bring nourishment to the hair follicle. The follicle is partly formed by the dermis and partly by the epidermis of the skin. At the bottom of the follicle there are finger-like projections, which contain connective tissue and the cells from which the new hair grows.

Attached to the hair at the underside is the erector muscle and the sebaceous gland which secretes a fatty substance—sebum. This consists of fatty acids, oleic oils, fats, hydrocarbons and steroids. It forms a thin film over the surface of the skin which gives shine to hair and keeps the skin soft and supple.

The hair is formed by a process of cell division, mitosis, around the root near the papilla. A healthy adult head contains about 150,000 hairs, varying in thickness and type according to the individual. Black hair is usually thicker than blond hair.

The hair grows roughly 1 mm to .04 mm per day. It is important to follow a good diet as this affects the growth and strength of the hair.

Hair is composed of an insoluble protein, keratin. It also contains a small amount of uric acid. The mineral content of hair varies according to the colour of the hair. For example, in

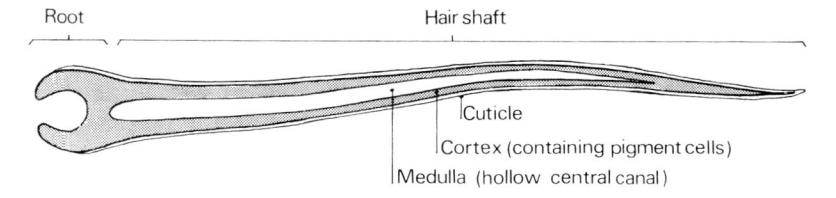

Fig. 14   Diagram of a hair.

brown hair there is carbon, nitrogen, hydrogen, phosphorus, sulphur and water. In red hair there is a much greater amount of iron than in any other colour. In all hair there is more carbon (44.3%) than any other of the substances.

The colour of the hair is inherited and it contains melanin and phenomelanin. Melanin is colourless, but it is acted upon by an enzyme, tyroninase, and becomes either a brown or a black pigment. Phenomelanin granules are red, brown and yellow. The hair can become grey due to copper deficiency due to the loss of the enzyme activity in the pigment cell. It can also become grey as a result of illness or shock.

2 HAIR DISEASES

Baldness or alopecia can be of several kinds. This can occur as a result of deficiency of diet, ill health or certain operations. Common baldness is not the same as these types, and accounts for most cases of baldness in men. In this condition the hair is lost gradually and usually starts at the crown and the temple. Very slight baldness shows a deep recession at the temple and, in older people, there is some loss of hair from the crown. If there is a great loss of hair the two areas join up and a state of advanced baldness is seen. Common baldness is usually inherited. It can be passed on by the female to her sons.

Dandruff is caused by skin irritation. It arises because the stratum corneum (the outer layer of the epidermis) sheds large scales, which are visible. This can be caused by excessive brushing or scratching, strong lotions and soft alkaline soaps applied to the hair. These can harm the skin and break down the outer layer of the epidermis. The second form of dandruff is due to a disease which causes large scales to fall on the shoulders. The more the head is scratched, the faster these scales are produced.

3 KEEPING THE HAIR HEALTHY

Wash the hair with mild shampoos, which are reinforced by active substances.

Treat the hair after shampooing with rinsing preparations and setting lotions in order to impart the gloss and firmness to it.

Groom the hair with hair conditioners in order to make it elastic and protect it from deterioration after frequent permanent waving.

Preserve the hair and its growth by constant attention, using hair lotions and hair treatment packs containing active substances.

4 HAIR PRODUCTS—SHAMPOOS, LOTIONS, HAIR DRESSINGS, DYES

A shampoo is a substance for removing dirt, grease and sweat from the hair. It should leave the hair shiny and in a good condition for setting.

In order to remove the grease, it is necessary to use a substance which has an affinity for grease—the surface active detergent materials. The detergent must allow the water to wet the hair fibre; it does this by reducing the surface tension of the water. Secondly, the interfacial tension must be reduced to an extent whereby the grease or dirt particles are displaced by the detergent solution. In selecting the detergent, the following properties must be noted:

1   the effect of the detergent on the surface to be cleaned;
2   the stability of the detergent, and
3   the efficiency of the detergent at an economic concentration.

Note: When choosing the detergent as a *shampoo base*, the following points should be taken into consideration:

1   The ease with which the shampoo can be spread all over the hair.
2   The lathering powers of the detergent, such as the volume of the lather, the speed with which the lather is formed and the stability of the lather in the hair.
3   The ease in rinsing the shampoo from the hair.
4   The colour and clarity of the shampoo.
5   The facility of combing wet hair after shampoo has been used.
6   The hair should shine after using the shampoo.
7   The speed at which the hair dries.

Modern shampoos are based on sulphated fatty alcohols and sulphonated fatty alcohol ethers.

Raw materials

Triethanolamine lauryl sulphate: This is a brown transparent viscous liquid. It is the basis of most liquid shampoos.

Alkyl sulphates: The alcohols are obtained by the reduction of the fatty acids. The alkyl sulphates are then obtained by the action of concentrated sulphuric acid (H_2SO_4) on the alcohol.

Sodium lauryl sulphate: This can be obtained either as a white or pale yellow powder which is highly soluble in water and is a good emulsifier; it may also be obtained as a paste.

Monoethanolamine lauryl sulphate: This is lighter in colour but very similar to triethanolamine lauryl sulphate. Its viscosity is increased by adding sodium chloride.

Turkey red oil (sulphated castor oil): This is a viscous water-miscible liquid which varies in colour from brown to yellow according to the quality of the castor oil from which it is made. It has detergent and emulsifying properties.

Cream shampoos

These cover every type from solid material to a soft cream. They can be made from a mixture of sodium lauryl sulphate and soap which makes the shampoo more viscous.

Liquid shampoos

These are stable and can be easily coloured and perfumed. The materials used are lauryl sulphate or lauryl ether sulphate. In addition there are the additives for foam and viscosity control such as the alkyl amides (coconut monoethanolamide) or lauric isopropanolamide. To control the viscosity, inorganic salts or the salts of organic bases are added. These can be small quantities of ammonium chloride or monoethanolamine hydrochloride. Egg, lanolin and lemon can also be added to the shampoo.

Lotion shampoos

These may be clear, opaque, or creamy liquids. A lotion shampoo has basically two main parts, (a) the active detergent which washes the hair, and (b) the opacifier which gives a pearly look to the shampoo and acts as an additive.

Formulae   *Grammes*

Cream shampoos

1	Sodium lauryl sulphate paste	25.0
	Stearic acid	6.5
	Lanolin	0.25
	Caustic soda	1.0
	Cetyl alcohol	0.5

Distilled water	67.75
Perfume	one to three drops
Preservative (Nipagin M)	one microspatula-full
Colour	one microspatula-full

Method:
1. Heat the stearic acid, sodium lauryl sulphate and lanolin and 80% of the water to 80°C.
2. Stir until homogeneous.
3. Heat the caustic soda and the remainder of the water (20%).
4. Add to (1) and stir for about 12–15 minutes.
   Add the perfume and colouring if required, at 40°C.

2. Manucol SS/LH

(Sodium alginate)	16.0
Sodium lauryl sulphate paste	30.0
Sodium chloride	4.0
Distilled water	50.0
Perfume	one to three drops
Colour	one microspatula-full
Preservative (Nipagin M)	one microspatula-full

Method:
1. Weigh all ingredients carefully.
2. Dissolve the manucol in water in a beaker (see Fig. 15).

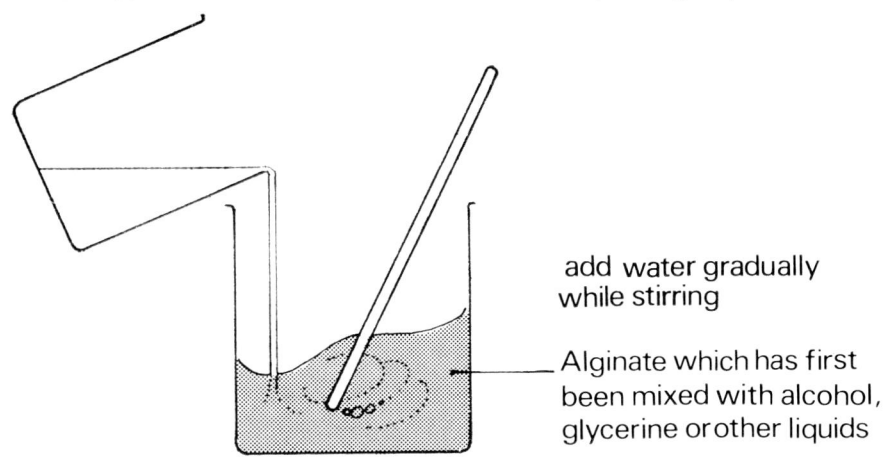

Fig. 15 Mixing sodium alginate (Manucol) with water. Stir the water, a little at first, into the powder to form a paste. Then add the remaining water. The formation of the paste is aided by first grinding the powder with a small quantity of the dispersing agent (e.g. glycerine, oils or alcohol) and then adding the water. Do not use hot water as this impairs the viscosity of the emulsion.

3 Mix the sodium chloride with the sulphonated lauryl paste in a mortar.
4 Heat the water solution to about 70°C.
5 Add the mixture of sodium chloride and sulphonated lauryl paste to the water with stirring. Allow to cool. Add the perfume, colour and preservative.

Note: The manucol is used as a thickener.

3   Sodium lauryl sulphate
        paste   25.0
     Diethylene glycol
        monostearate   2.0
     Sodium hydroxide   0.75
     Stearic acid   5.0
     Distilled water   67.25
     Perfume   one to three drops
     Colour   one microspatula-full
     Preservative (Nipagin M)   one microspatula-full

Method:
1 Dissolve the sodium hydroxide in the water then heat to 70°C.
2 Heat the remainder of the ingredients, excluding the perfume and colour, to 70°C. Then add to the sodium hydroxide solution.
3 Stir until cool.
4 Add the perfume and colour after the emulsion had been cooled down to 45°C.

4   Sodium lauryl sulphate
        paste   25.0
     Stearic acid   7.0
     Sodium hydroxide
        (as a solid)   1.0
     Distilled water   67.0
     Preservative (Nipagin M)   one microspatula-full
     Perfume   one to three drops

Method:
1 Heat the sodium lauryl sulphate paste, stearic acid and half the water in a beaker, to give a smooth liquid free from lumps. (70°C)
2 Dissolve the sodium hydroxide and preservative in the remaining water (70°C).
3 Add (2) to (1) with constant stirring until a smooth homogeneous mixture has been obtained, and then allow to cool. Add the perfume when the temperature has fallen to 35°C.

5   Sodium lauryl sulphate
       paste   50.0
    Stearic acid   7.0
    Sodium hydroxide   1.0
    Preservative (Nipagin M)   one microspatula-full
    Perfume   one to three drops
    Distilled water   42.0
Method: As above.

6 *a* Sodium lauryl sulphate
         paste   50.0
      Isopropanolamide   3.0
      Stearic acid   7.0
   b Sodium hydroxide   1.0
      Distilled water   39.0
      Preservative (Nipagin M)   one microspatula-full
   c Perfume   one to three drops
Method: Heat (*a*) to 70°C. Heat (*b*) to 70°C. Add (*b*) to (*a*). Stir until an emulsion is formed. Add the perfume at 35°C.

7   *Liquid Cream Shampoo*
    Sodium lauryl sulphate
       paste   25.0
    Polyethylene glycol
       monostearate   5.0
    Magnesium stearate   2.0
    Oleyl alcohol   one to three drops
    Manucol SS44   one microspatula-full
    Distilled water   68.0
    Perfume   one to three drops
    Preservative (Nipagin M)   one microspatula-full
Method:
  1 Mix the magnesium stearate with the sodium lauryl sulphate paste.
  2 Add the polyethylene glycol monostearate to the water and stir. Then add the oleyl alcohol. Heat the mixture to 75°C.
  3 Add the water to this with constant stirring.
  4 Add the perfume and preservative at 40°C.

8   *Anti-Dandruff Cream*
    Sodium lauryl sulphate
       paste   25.0
    Stearic acid   7.0
    Sodium hydroxide   1.0
    Biosulphur powder   2.0
    Distilled water   65.0
    Preservative (Nipagin M)   one microspatula-full
    Perfume   one drop

Method: Dissolve the sodium hydroxide in water with heating (75°C). Add the biosulphur to the sodium hydroxide solution. Mix the stearic acid and sodium lauryl sulphate paste and warm slightly to about 60°C. Add to the aqueous solution. Stir until cool. Add the perfume and preservative.

Liquid Shampoos

1
a	Triethanolamine lauryl sulphate	45.0
b	Empilan CME (coconut monoethanolamide)	2.0
c	Distilled water	53.0
d	Perfume	one to three drops
e	Preservative (Nipagin M)	one microspatula-full

Method: Heat (a) and (b) to about 65°C. Heat (c) and (e) to about 65°C. Mix together. Add (d) when cool.

2
a	Triethanolamine lauryl sulphate	40.0
b	Preservative (Nipagin M)	0.2
c	Distilled water	59.8
d	Colour (if desired)	one microspatula-full
e	Perfume	one to three drops

Method: Add (b) to (c). Add colour (d). Then mix with (a). Add (e).

3
Triethanolamine lauryl sulphate	30.0
Sulphated castor oil	5.0
Toilet spirit	20.0
Distilled water	45.0
Perfume	one drop
Preservative (Nipagin M)	one microspatula-full

Method: Dissolve the castor oil in the toilet spirit. Add the lauryl sulphate, then add the water, preservative and perfume.

4
a	Triethanolamine lauryl sulphate	40.0
b	Empilan CME	3.2
c	Distilled water	56.8
d	Perfume	one drop
e	Preservative (Nipagin M)	one microspatula-full

Method: Heat (a) and (b) to about 65°C. Heat (c) and (e) to about 65°C. Mix together. Add (d) when cool.

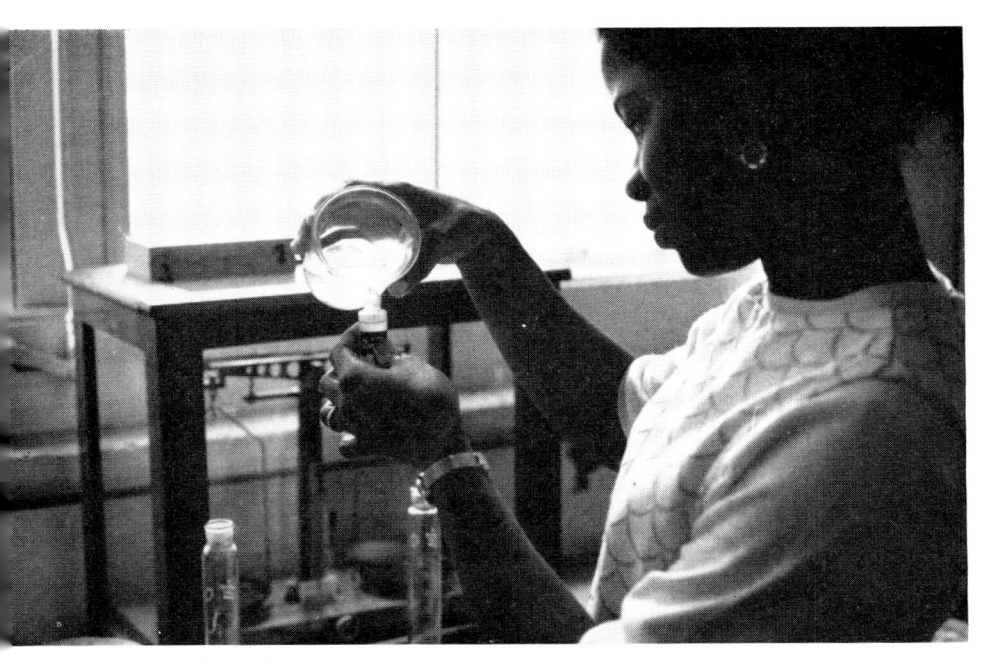

Fig. 16 Lotion shampoo.

Lotion shampoos

1. Sodium lauryl sulphate
    paste   16.0
    Empicol ESB 30   20.0
    Ethylene glycol
     monostearate   2.4
    Empilan CDE
     (coconut diethanolamide)   4.0
    Distilled water   57.6
    Preservative (Nipagin M)   one microspatula-full
    Perfume   one to three drops

Method: Heat all the ingredients (with the exception of the perfume) together at 65°–70°C to give a smooth liquid free from lumps. Allow to cool with slow stirring Add the perfume at 35°C.

2. Sodium lauryl ether sulphate
    (liquid)   40.0
    Ethylene glycol
     monostearate   2.0
    Empilan CDE   5.0

Stearic acid	1.0
Sodium chloride	0.4
Distilled water	51.6
Preservative (Nipagin M)	0.2
Perfume	one to three drops

Method: As above.

3 *Liquid Soapless Shampoo*

a Triethanolamine lauryl sulphate	50.0
b Distilled water	50.0
c Perfume	one to three drops
d Colour (water-soluble dye)	one microspatula-full
e Preservative (Nipagin M)	one microspatula-full

Method: Mix (a), (b) and (e) together (without too much agitation) in a measuring cylinder. Add (c) and (d), and stir.

4 *Clear Liquid Shampoo* (contains a foam stabilizer)

a Empicol TL (HO)	50.0
b Preservative (Nipagin M)	one microspatula-full
c Distilled water	50.0
d Perfume	one to three drops

Method: Dissolve (a) in (c). Add (b). Mix thoroughly, then add perfume.

5 a Sodium lauryl ether sulphate	60.0
b Preservative (Nipagin M)	one microspatula-full
c Distilled water	40.0
d Perfume	one to three drops

Method: As above.

Jelly shampoos

These consist of a lauryl sulphate thickened by an alkaline sulphate, Empicol.

1

Sodium lauryl sulphate paste	47.0
Oleic acid	20.0
Triethanolamine	10.5
Distilled water	22.5
Preservative (Nipagin M)	one microspatula-full
Perfume	one or two drops
Empilan GMS	one microspatula-full

Method: Mix water, oleic acid and sodium lauryl sulphate; heat to 60°C. Add the triethanolamine slowly with stirring. Pour into a container and allow to cool. Add the perfume at 35°C.

2   Empicol ESB 30 (or ESB 3)   69.0
    Empilan CME   4.0
    Empilan LDE   2.0
    Sodium chloride   one microspatula-full
    Preservative (Nipagin M)   one microspatula-full
    Distilled water   25.0
    Perfume   one or two drops

Method: Heat all ingredients together with stirring until a clear homogeneous liquid is formed. Allow to cool.

3   Empicol ESB 30 (or ESB 3)   50.0
    Empilan CME   4.0
    Empilan LDE   2.0
    Sodium chloride   one microspatula-full
    Preservative (Nipagin M)   one microspatula-full
    Distilled water   44.0
    Perfume   one or two drops

Method: As above.

Hair Setting Lotions

1   Toilet spirit   10.0
    Glycerine   5.0
    Gum tragacanth   1.2
    Distilled water   83.8
    Preservative (Nipagin M)   one microspatula-full
    Colour   one microspatula-full

Method: Grind the gum tragacanth with water in a mortar. Add the glycerine and toilet spirit, perfume and colour.

2   Manutex AKP   1.0
    Toilet spirit   5.0
    Glycerine   1.0
    Preservative (Nipagin M)   0.1
    Distilled water   92.9
    Colour   one microspatula-full
    Perfume   one drop

Method: Disperse the Manutex and preservative in the toilet spirit and glycerine. Heat water to 60°C. Add with stirring. The colour and perfume are then added.

Hair Creams

1 a Beeswax   1.5
    Oleic acid   1.0
    Petroleum jelly   39.6
  b Calcium hydroxide   0.07
  c Magnesium sulphate
    (to stabilise)   2.0

  d Distilled water   55.83
  e Perfume   one drop
   Preservative (Nipagin M)   one microspatula-full

Method: Heat (*a*) in a beaker to 70–72°C. Dissolve (*b*) and (*c*) in (*d*) by heating to 70°–72°C. Add this solution to the oil phase. Add the perfume and preservative at 42°C. Continue to stir down until cool.

2 *a* Petroleum jelly   6.0
  Mineral oil   35.0
  Wheat germ oil   2.5
  Lanolin anhydrous   3.0
  Beeswax   12.0
  Sorbitan monolaurate   1.0
  Sorbitan sesquioleate   3.0
  Polyoxethene sorbitan
   monolaurate   2.0
 b Borax   0.5
  Distilled water   35.0
  Preservative (Nipagin M)   one microspatula-full
 c Perfume   one or two drops

Method: Heat (*a*) to 70°C. Heat (*b*) to 72°C. Add (*b*) to (*a*). Add (*c*) at 42°C. Stir until cold.

3 *a* Mineral oil   30.0
  Lanette wax SX   3.0
 b Distilled water   67.0
  Preservative (Nipagin M)   one microspatula-full
 c Perfume   one or two drops

Method: Heat (*a*) to 70°C. Heat (*b*) to 72°C. Add (*b*) to (*a*) and stir. Add the perfume at 30°C.

4 *a* Mineral oil   33.2
  Beeswax   3.0
  Stearic acid   0.5
  Cetyl alcohol   1.3
 b Distilled water   60.0
  Borax   one microspatula-full
  Triethanolamine   2.0
  Preservative (Nipagin M)   one microspatula-full
 c Perfume   one or two drops

Method: Heat (*a*) and (*b*) independently to 65°C. Add (*a*) to (*b*) with constant stirring. Add the perfume at 35°C.

5 *a* Mineral oil   38.0
  Beeswax   1.5
  Stearic acid   0.5

b	Limewater	60.0
	Perfume	one or two drops
	Preservative (Nipagin M)	one microspoatla-full

Method: Heat (*a*) to 70°C. Heat (*b*) to 20°C. Add (*b*) to (*a*) quickly with rapid stirring.

6   *Medicated Hair Cream*
a	Collone QAC	5.0
	Beeswax	3.0
	Light liquid paraffin	20.0
b	Distilled water	72.0
	Preservative (Nipagin M)	one microsatula-full
c	Perfume	one or two drops

Method: Heat (*a*) and (*b*) independently to 70°C. Add (*b*) to (*a*). Add the perfume when cool.

7   *Hair Conditioning Cream*
a	Collone QAC	10.0
	Lanolin	3.0
b	Distilled water	87.0
	Preservative (Nipagin M)	one microspatula-full
c	Perfume	one or two drops

Method: As above.

8   *Hairdressing Cream, clear*
Lanolin	15.0
Distilled water	85.0
Preservative (Nipagin M)	one microspatula-full
Perfume	one to three drops

Method:
1 Heat lanolin to 70°C.
2 Heat water and preservative to 72°C. Add (2) to (1). Stir to form an emulsion. Add the perfume at 50°C.

9   *Hair Conditioning Cream*
a	Lanette wax SX	15.0
	Lecithin	0.5
	Cholesterol	0.5
	Olive oil	5.0
b	Lemon juice or citric acid	1.0
c	Distilled water	78.0
	Preservative (Nipagin M)	one microspatula-full
d	Perfume (lemon cologne)	one to three drops

Method: Heat (*a*) in a beaker to 70°C. Heat (*c*) to 70°C. Add (*c*) to (*a*). Stir, add the perfume at 35°C. Add the lemon juice.

10 *Hair Conditioning Cream*
   a Lanette wax SV   15.0
     Lanolin   3.0
   b Citric acid or lemon juice   1.0
   c Distilled water   81.0
     Preservative (Nipagin M)   one microspatula-full
   d Perfume (lemon cologne)   one to three drops

Method: As above.

11 *Hair Cream*
   a Petroleum jelly   10.0
     Mineral oil   30.0
     Polyethylene glycol 400
       monostearate   4.0
     Abracol SPA (emulsifier)   5.0
   b Distilled water   51.0
     Preservative (Nipagin M)   one microspatula-full
   c Perfume   one to three drops

Method: Heat (*a*) and (*b*) independently to 75°C. Add (*b*) to (*a*) slowly with stirring. Perfume at 45°C.

12 *Hair Dressing Cream*
   a Mineral oil   37.5
     Lanolin   3.0
     White petroleum jelly   7.5
     Beeswax   2.0
     Zinc stearate   1.0
     Arlacel 83   3.0
   b Borax   0.5
     Distilled water   45.5
     Preservative (Nipagin M)   one microspatula-full
   c Perfume   one to three drops

Method: Heat (*a*) to 75°C. Heat (*b*) to 77°C. Add (*b*) to (*a*) slowly with stirring. Perfume at 45°C.

13 *Brilliantine*
     Isopropyl myristate   24.0
     Lanolin   1.0
     Mineral oil (wheat germ oil)   55.0
     Sesame or sunflower oil   20.0
     Colour   one microspatula-full
     Perfume   one or two drops
     Antioxidant (Progallon)   one drop
     Preservative (Nipagin M)   one microspatula-full

Method: Melt (70°C) all oils and waxes together in a beaker. Add the preservative, antioxidant, colour and perfume.

14 Spirit Brilliantine

Isopropyl myristate	20.0
Cetyl alcohol	2.0
Toilet spirit	78.0
Colour	one microspatula-full
Perfume	three to five drops
Preservative (Nipagin M)	one microspatula-full

Method: Mix all the ingredients together in a measuring cylinder or beaker.

Solid Brilliantine

15
Petroleum jelly	90.0
Paraffin wax	10.0
Colour	one microspatula-full
Preservative (Nipagin M)	one microspatula-full
Perfume	one to three drops

Method: Melt (70°C) the waxes in a beaker. Add the colour, perfume and preservative.

16
Carnauba wax	5.0
Wheat germ oil	20.0
Petroleum jelly	70.0
Paraffin wax	5.0
Colour	one microspatula-full
Perfume	one drop
Preservative (Nipagin M)	one microspatula-full

Method: As above.

17
Mineral oil	85.0
Isopropyl myristate	15.0
Perfume	one to three drops
Preservative (Nipagin M)	one microspatula-full

Method: Mix the perfume with the isopropyl myristate and mineral oil, in a beaker. Add preservative. Strain through silk or fine muslin into another beaker.

18
Mineral oil	75.0
Acetoglyceride L/C	10.0
Isopropyl myristate	15.0
Perfume	one to three drops
Preservative (Nipagin M)	one microspatula-full

Method: Mix all ingredients together in a beaker, and strain through silk or fine muslin into another beaker.

Dyes

These are now used extensively by men and women of all ages.

Great care should be taken in preparing this type of cosmetic. It is important that the dye should not injure the hair shaft and that it should colour only the shaft, while retaining the natural gloss of the hair. It should have no toxic effect on the skin and hair, and no irritating effect on the scalp. It should be stable on exposure to air, sunlight and salt water. Before applying hair dyes it is most important to remove all grease from the hair.

The hair dyes are divided into three main groups—metallic dyes, vegetable dyes and synthetic dyes.

Metallic dyes: The most commonly used are salts of lead (e.g. lead acetate), bismuth (e.g. ammoniacal bismuth citrate) and silver (e.g. ammoniacal silver nitrate). Copper, nickel and cobalt salts can also be used in some cases.

Vegetable dyes: The most widely used is henna. Henna is composed of dried powdered leaves of plants. Its hair dyeing properties are due to the presence of lawsone, which is soluble in hot water. Henna is not an irritant.

Synthetic dyes: e.g. D & C orange No. 4, D & C black, D & C brown.

Pyrogallic acid: This is a very important raw material used in dyes. It occurs in fine white crystals. It is necessary to add an alkali to hasten oxidation.

Paraphenylenediamine: This is the most important hair dye used. It occurs as white crystals and is used with either hydrogen peroxide or potassium dichromate.

Formulae   *Grammes*

1   *Henna Dye*
    Powdered henna   72.0
    Pyrogallic acid   12.0
    Copper sulphate (powder) 8.0
    Colour (burnt senna)   8.0
    Distilled water (enough to make a paste)

Method: Make into a paste with hot water (62°–75°C) when required.

2   *Henna Dye (liquid)*
    Copper chloride   4.0
    Pyrogallic acid   2.0
    Distilled water   90.0
    Toilet spirit   4.0

Method: Dissolve the copper chloride and pyrogallic acid in the water. Add the toilet spirit.

3   *Silver dye*
    Solution A
    Distilled water   58.0
    Toilet spirit   40.0
    Pyrogallic acid   2.0

    Solution B
    (i) *Brown dye*
    Silver nitrate   1.0
    Dilute ammonia (10% or less) 6.0 cm^3
    Distilled water   100.0

    (ii) *Ash Blond dye*
    Silver nitrate   1.0
    Dilute ammonia (10% or less) 4.5 cm^3
    Distilled water   100.0

    Solution C
    Distilled water   100.0
    Sodium thiosulphate   2.0

Method: Mix the ingredients of each solution independently in glass beakers. Store in dark bottle.

To dye the hair:

1. Rinse with Solution A.
2. Rinse with Solution B(i) or (ii) according to colour required.
3. Allow 15 minutes for Solution B to develop, then rinse with Solution C. Do not wash the hair for a few hours.

4   *Lead Acetate dye*
    Lead acetate   6.0
    Sodium thiosulphate   1.2
    Glycerine   8.2
    Toilet spirit   10.0 cm^3
    Rose water   80.0 cm^3

Method: Dissolve the lead acetate in 10 cm^3 of rose water. Mix the remaining liquids together and dissolve the sodium thiosulphate in this mixture. Pour the sodium thiosulphate solution into the lead acetate solution. A precipitate will form which will then dissolve. Pour this solution into brown bottles *immediately*. Add one or two drops of ether, to remove the air from the bottle and cork securely.

   Synthetic Organic Dyes
5 *Auburn rinse*
   D & C Orange No. 4
      (colour)   4.5
   Tartaric acid   93.0

	FD & C Red No. 1	2.5

Method : Dissolve all the ingredients in water.

6   *Black rinse*

	D & C Black No. 1	16.0
	D & C Red No. 1	2.4
	D & C Brown No. 1	1.6
	Tartaric acid	80.0

Method : Dissolve all the ingredients in water.

5 STRUCTURE OF NAILS

Nails consist of protective translucent plates covering the top surfaces of the last bone joint of each finger. They are composed of horny epidermal cells which, instead of being shed

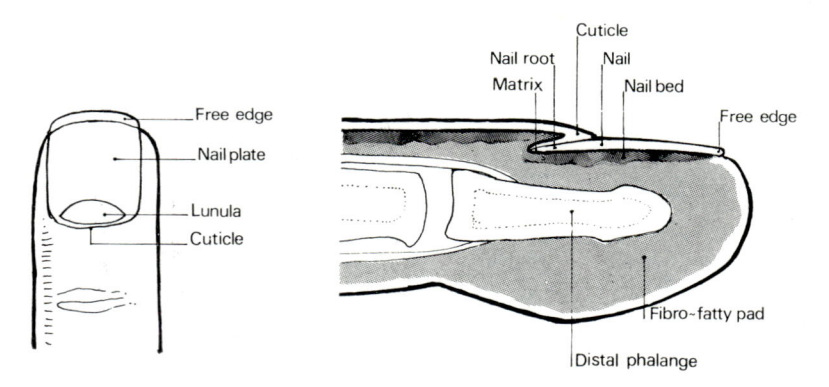

Fig. 17   Diagrams of a human nail.

separately in the form of flakes (as in the case of skin), are first built up into a definite protective structure.

The nail is composed of (a) the nail plate, and (b) the nail bed upon which it rests.

The nail grows towards its free edge and away from the matrix or growth portion of the nail. This matrix is the most important part of the nail and is composed of cells similar to the malpighian layer of the skin.

The most important constituent of the nail is keratin, which is a protein containing a large amount of sulphur.

The nail bed plays an important part in the nutrition of the nail itself. If the nail is separated from the nail bed by injury, it becomes discoloured. Nails are harmed by detergents and by using too much lacquer.

The half moon occurs at the base of the nail, under the nail plate. The nail grows at the rate of 3 mm per month. If there are furrows running across each nail, they mark dates of illnesses. White spots on nails are due to the presence of keratohyatin granules or enlarged acid cells. The moisture content of the nails is about 0.15–0.76.

6 NAIL CARE

1   Remove all traces of old enamel.
2   Shape the nails with emery board. File from the side towards the centre. Shape the nails in an oval and allow them to extend about one-sixteenth of an inch from the edge of the finger. In this way the nail is less liable to break and split.
3   Massage nail cream into the cuticles and around the sides of the finger tips.
4   Soak the hands in warm soapy water for a few minutes, rinse and dry.
5   Apply cuticle remover and push the cuticles back with orange stick. Use orange stick to clean under the nails, then scrub the nails with a nail brush in warm soapy water.
6   Trim any rough edges on cuticles, then wash the hands and apply good moisture cream or lotion.
7   Clean the nails with enamel remover, then apply the enamel.
8   Apply a base coat of enamel, then, when dry, apply a second, and perhaps a third coat.

To preserve the nails it is essential to follow a sensible diet and to get adequate rest. A good diet and plenty of sleep will benefit the strength and appearance of the nails. To encourage long nails, apply a cuticle massage cream. Avoid hard knocks or bruises to the nails.

Formulae   *Grammes*

1   *Cuticle Remover*
    Potassium hydroxide   2.0
    Glycerine   20.0
    Distilled water   78.0
    Perfume   one to three drops
    Preservative (Nipagin M) one microspatula-full

Method: Dissolve the potassium hydroxide in glycerine

and water in a beaker. Add the perfume and preservative.

> *Note:* Potassium hydroxide is a caustic substance. If it is allowed to come in contact with the skin the affected area should be washed immediately with plenty of cold water. Do not leave pellets or flakes lying around. Replace the stopper in the bottle immediately after use.

2   Cuticle Cream
    Soft paraffin   40.0
    Spermaceti   20.0
    Lanolin   40.0
    Perfume   one to three drops
    Preservative (Nipagin M)   one microspatula-full

Method: Melt all the ingredients (with the exception of the perfume) together in a beaker. Add the perfume when cooled down to 35°C.

3   Cuticle Cream
    Beeswax   1.0
    Petroleum jelly   95.0
    Emulsene 1219   4.0
    Perfume   one drop
    Preservative (Nipagin M)   one microspatula-full

Method: As above.

4   Cuticle Cream
    Lanolin   4.0
    Liquid paraffin   50.0
    Beeswax   16.0
    Borax   1.0
    Emulsifier   5.0
    Distilled water   24.0
    Perfume   one to three drops
    Preservative (Nipagin M)   one microspatula-full

Method:
  1 Melt all waxes and oils together to 75°C.
  2 Heat the water to 75°C. Add the preservative to the water. Add (2) to (1). Stir down to 25–35°C. Add the perfume.

5   Nail Cream
    Beeswax   15.0
    Ozokerite   2.5
    Montan wax   2.5
    Mineral oil   40.0
    Cetyl alcohol   2.0
    Borax   1.5

Aluminium stearate	10.0
Distilled water	26.5
Perfume	one drop
Preservative (Nipagin M)	one microspatula-full

Method:

1 Melt all waxes and oils in a beaker. (75°C).

2 Heat the water and preservative. (75°C). Add (2) to (1). Mix in the aluminium stearate. Add the perfume.

6 *Nail Bleach*
| Orange flower water | 95.0 |
| Citric acid or lemon juice | 5.0 |

Method: Mix all the ingredients together.

7 *Nail Bleach*
Glycerine	10.0
Rose water	40.0
Hydrogen peroxide (5 vol.)	50.0

Method: Mix all the ingredients together.

8 *Nail Varnish Remover*
Acetone	98.0
Glycerine	2.0
Perfume	one to three drops

Method: Mix all the ingredients together.

7 TEETH (See Fig. 18, p. 114.)

Man has 32 teeth altogether (16 in each of the upper and lower jaws). In each jaw there are 4 incisor, 2 canine, 4 premolar and 4 molar teeth. These, if removed or damaged, are not replaced after the "permanent" teeth have replaced the "milk" teeth in the front of the mouth. Damage may be caused by allowing food particles to remain lodged in the teeth. The particles may chemically attack the enamel and dentine, causing holes to appear, and eventually causing the tooth to decay. Such food particles should, therefore, be regularly brushed away. Toothpaste is a valuable aid to cleaning the teeth.

8 TOOTHPASTE

A toothpaste is composed of:

1 a polishing agent,

2 a humectant (moistener),

3 a detergent and foaming agent,

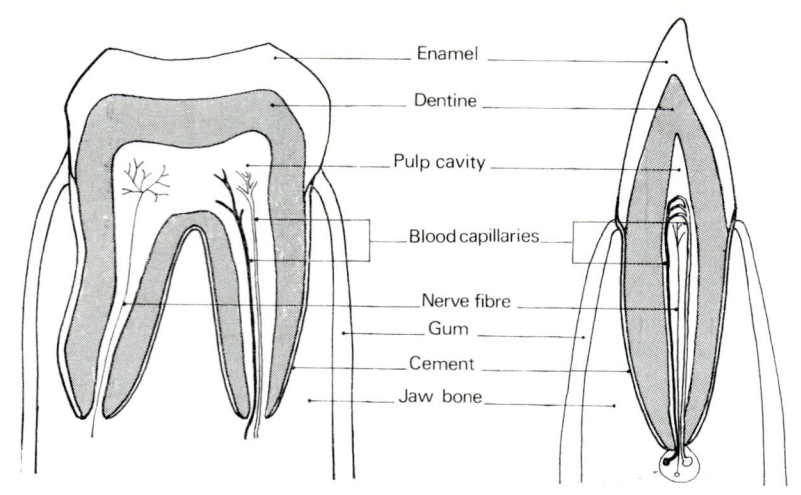

*Fig. 18   Teeth. There are two types of teeth, the simple or conical ones and more complex ones, which have their upper surfaces broadened into crowns for crushing and chewing purposes. Both types have the same basic construction. On the outside there is a layer of **enamel**, which is hard and shiny. The bulk of the tooth consists of **dentine**, which is similar in chemical composition to bone. Inside this there is the **pulp cavity**, which contains soft materials, including blood vessels and nerves.*

    4 a binding agent,
    5 a sweetener,
    6 a flavour,
    7 a preservative.

1   Polishing agent: This is one of the most important ingredients of a toothpaste, as it is responsible for removing particles of food which have become lodged in the teeth. It also helps to remove any discoloration from the teeth. It is usually about half the total weight of the toothpaste. The materials mostly used can be chosen from the following: precipitated chalk, tricalcium phosphate, aluminium sulphate, magnesium trisilicate.

2   Humectant—Moistener: This is usually added to the toothpaste to prevent drying out and hardening of the paste. The materials mostly used are glycerine, sorbitol, propylene glycol. The best one to use is glycerine, as it easily makes a non-drying paste.

3 The detergent and foaming agent: A detergent is put into the toothpaste to aid the action of the polishing agent by wetting the teeth and any particles of food, and also to emulsify the mucus. The amount of detergent needed varies from between 1.5% to 5% of the total weight of the toothpaste. Soap has been superseded by soapless detergents because of the improved foam and better taste. The most suitable and popular types of detergent ingredients used are sodium lauryl sulphate or magnesium lauryl sulphate.

4 The binding agent: This is most essential in order to prevent the separation of the toothpaste. The gums mostly used are:

- a Starch
- b Gum tragacanth
- c Sodium alginate (Manucol SA)
- d Modified Irish moss (this is very good and gives a very stable toothpaste), and
- e Synthetics such as polyethylene glycols.

5 The sweetener: Saccharine is used at concentrations of 0.1–1.3%. Sugar can also be used, but it tends to crystallize.

6 The flavouring: The most widely used is oil of peppermint.

7 Preservatives: A non-toxic preservative is used such as sodium benzoate or sodium hydroxybenzoate.

General method of preparation

1 The binding agents are dispersed in the humectant (moistener).

2 The detergent is then added very slowly in order to prevent foaming difficulties.

3 The water and preservative is then added to the mixture.

4 The sweetener and the polishing agent are then mixed in and thoroughly stirred to give a smooth paste.

5 The flavouring is then added and incorporated into the mixture.

Formulae   *Grammes*

Toothpastes

1	Precipitated chalk	57.0
	Sodium lauryl sulphate	1.0
	Glycerine	21.0

	Gum tragacanth	1.5
	Flavouring	one drop
	Saccharine	one drop
	Distilled water	19.5
	Preservative	
	(Sodium benzoate)	one microspatula-full
2	Precipitated chalk	45.0
	Gum tragacanth	0.5
	Sodium palmitate	7.0
	Glycerine	20.0
	Neutral sodium silicate	1.0
	Flavouring	one drop
	Saccharine	one drop
	Distilled water	26.5
	Preservative	
	(Sodium benzoate)	one microspatula-full
3	Gum tragacanth	1.0
	Propylene glycol	17.0
	Glycerine	8.5
	Sodium lauryl sulphate	3.65
	Dicalcium phosphate	51.0
	Flavouring	1.1
	Saccharine solution	0.85
	Distilled water	17.0
	Preservative	
	(Sodium benzoate)	one microspatula-full
4	Sodium alginate	1.0
	Propylene glycol	17.0
	Glycerine	8.4
	Sodium lauryl sulphate	3.0
	Precipitated chalk	40.0
	Flavouring	1.7
	Saccharine solution	0.63
	Distilled water	28.0
	Preservative	
	(Sodium benzoate)	0.27
5	Precipitated chalk	44.0
	Magnesium carbonate	1.0
	Magnesium hydroxide	3.5
	Sodium lauryl sulphate	1.0
	Gum tragacanth	1.0
	Glycerine	30.0
	Oil of peppermint	1.0
	Saccharine	0.1

	Distilled water	18.4
	Preservative (Sodium benzoate)	one microspatula-full

Tooth Powders

1	Precipitated calcium carbonate	95.0
	Dental soap	5.0
	Flavouring	one drop
	Saccharine	one drop
2	Sodium bicarbonate	4.0
	Precipitated chalk	90.0
	White powdered Castile soap	6.0
	Oil of peppermint	one drop
	Oil of cloves	one drop
	Oil of cinnamon	one drop

7
Cosmetics for the drama group

A different range of cosmetics is needed for the stage, because stage lighting bleaches the natural colours of the actor or actress. This bleaching effect can be counteracted by using grease paint, which has had the correct colours blended into it. This corrective use of colours applies equally to the other range of cosmetics used for stage make-up, such as powders, lipsticks and eye shadows. The colours are numbered 1, $1\frac{1}{2}$, 2, 3, 4 and so on to 20.

1 GREASEPAINT

A greasepaint is composed of two distinct parts blended together—the fat base and the dry base. It should have the following properties: The paint should not be too hard, too oily or too fatty. It should be easily applied, should spread well and have a good covering power.

1 The fat base: This can be chosen from a fairly wide range, including almond oil, mineral oil, liquid paraffin, white petroleum jelly, beeswax and ceresine. Hard paraffin wax and lanolin lard can sometimes be used, but these have a strong smell and are only used in very cheap products.

2 The dry base: A suitable base can be used from a choice of the following powders—titanium dioxide (cosmetic quality), precipitated chalk, kaolin, zinc oxide, magnesium stearate, magnesium carbonate, satinex, talc.

Formulae for making a greasepaint

Fat base (This can be chosen from any of the following formulae.)

		Grammes
1	Lanolin (anhydrous)	5.0
	Ceresine (white)	25.0
	Mineral oil	70.0
	Preservative	
	(Nipagin M or Nipasol M)	one microspatula-full
2	Almond oil	34.0
	Petroleum jelly	30.0
	Paraffin wax	30.0

	Beeswax (white)	6.0
	Preservative	
	(Nipagin M or Nipasol M)	one microspatula-full
3	Lanolin	5.0
	Mineral oil	70.0
	Beeswax (white)	25.0
	Perfume	one drop
	Preservative	
	(Nipagin M or Nipasol M)	one microspatula-full

Dry base (This can be chosen from any of the following formulae.)

1	Kaolin	5.0
	Zinc oxide	70.0
	Satinex	5.0
	Precipitated chalk	20.0
2	Zinc stearate	2.0
	Titanium dioxide	5.0
	Magnesium carbonate (light)	5.0
	Zinc oxide	10.0
	Calcium carbonate	20.0
	Talc	58.0
3	Zinc oxide	70.0
	Titanium dioxide	20.0
	Talc	10.0

Method:
(*a*) Melt the fats together in a beaker. Add preservative, strain through fine muslin and add the perfume when cool (35°C).

(*b*) Mix the powders in a mortar and pestle. Pass through a sieve (very fine). If this is not easily obtained, a nylon stocking can be placed on a large evaporating dish and the powder sieved this way.

Note: Half the above quantities can be used if smaller amounts are required.

Formulae for making a white greasepaint

	Grammes
Dry Base	55.0
Fat Base	45.0

Method: Heat very gently to 75°C the fat base in a beaker. Add the sifted powder. Mix the two bases together over a water bath. While the mixture is still molten pass it through a piece of fine muslin, silk or nylon, then run the mixture into moulds (a lipstick mould is quite suitable, but gives very small sticks). When the greasepaint has set, remove from the mould and wrap some silver foil around the end. The greasepaint can also be poured into jars instead of being moulded.

To make the coloured greasepaint, the dry base is mixed with the appropriate colour and then it is added to the fat base, and the procedure is followed as in the preparation of the white greasepaint. The usual colours required are flesh colour, suntan and pale pink. If a blue greasepaint is required, the following colours are mixed together: blue (cobalt), ultramarine and mauve.

Reds, Nos. 1, 2 and 3 are made by mixing a deep scarlet and carmine, e.g.

	Grammes
Fat base	80.0
Colour scarlet	10.0
Carmine lake	10.0

For black colours, lamp black is added to the fat base:

	Grammes
Carbon black	20.0
Fat base	80.0

Method: Melt the fat base. Add lamp black. Mix thoroughly and pour into jars.

If a harder type of black paint is required, the fat base should consist of the following:

	Grammes
Hard paraffin	40.0
White petroleum jelly	42.0
Lamp black	18.0

Method: Melt the waxes. Add the lamp black. Stir. Pour into moulds. When set, remove and wrap either cellophane or silver foil around the ends.

2 MIXING OF COLOURS

It is necessary to mix colours in various proportions to obtain the correct shade, as for example, flesh tones. The colours should be mixed as follows: red and yellow, carmine and scarlet; for a more yellowish tint, golden ochre and yellow, and other shades of yellow.

For flesh colours from No. 3 upwards, the following colours are mixed together:

	Grammes
Burnt sienna	1.0
Golden ochre	15.0
Crimson lakes	2.0
	18.0

For 100 g of dry base, add to it the 18 g of colour. Then add this mixture to the fat base. This makes a very dark greasepaint suitable for a soldier or sailor.

For No. 1, add to 100 g base, 0.5 g of the colour.

For No. $1\frac{1}{2}$, add to 100 g base, 1.0 g of the colour.

For No. 2, add to 100 g base, 5.0 g of the colour.

For No. 3, add to 100 g base, 8.0 g of the colour.

To make No. 4 colour, mix golden ochre (5 g) and Armenian Bol (18 g). This is then added to the mixture of dry and fat base, which has been mixed using a mortar and pestle.

To make No. 5, mix the following:

	Grammes
Yellow ochre	15.0
Burnt sienna	3.0
Geranium	2.0

and add to the base, as previously explained.

3 REMOVAL OF STAGE MAKE UP

For the removal of stage make-up, greasepaint remover and a very fatty cold cream are used. The base used for the cold cream is usually lard, with the addition of spermaceti, ceresine, cocoa butter and mineral oil.

Formulae *Grammes*

Cold creams

1	Lard	80.0
	Cocoa butter	20.0
	Perfume	one to three drops
	Preservative (Nipagin M)	one microspatula-full
2	Lard	80.0
	Spermaceti	20.0

	Perfume	one to three drops
	Preservative (Nipagin M)	one microspatula-full
3	Lard	80.0
	Ceresine	20.0
	Perfume	one to three drops
	Preservative (Nipagin M)	one microspatula-full

Method: Melt waxes (75°C). Add perfume and preservative. Pour into tins.

Greasepaint remover

1	White petroleum jelly	62.0
	Ceresine	37.5
	Perfume	0.5
	Preservative (Nipagin M)	one microspatula-full

Method: Melt the fats (70°–75°C), add the perfume and preservative and pour into a mould.

2	White petroleum jelly	80.0
	Beeswax, white	5.0
	Mineral oil	15.0
	Perfume	one to five drops
	Preservative (Nipagin M)	one microspatula-full

Method: Melt the waxes (75°C). Add the perfume and preservative. Pour into jars.

Rouges

1	Beeswax	62.5
	Zinc oxide	35.7
	Petroleum jelly	1.8
	Colour	one microspatula-full
	Perfume	one to three drops
	Preservative (Nipagin M)	one microspatula-full

Method:
  1 Melt the beeswax and petroleum jelly in a beaker (75°C).
  2 Add the colour to the zinc oxide and perfume. Add (2) to (1).

2	Petroleum jelly	89.0
	Ceresine wax	11.0
	Colour (as required)	one microspatula-full
	Preservative (Nipagin M)	one microspatula-full
	Perfume	one to three drops

Method:
  1 Melt (70°C) a little of the petroleum jelly in a beaker. Add colour and mix thoroughly.

2 Heat the remaining petroleum jelly and ceresine wax to 70°C. Then add to (1). Blend together in a mortar.

3 a Lanolin 5.0
Cocoa butter 5.0
Beeswax 14.0
Liquid paraffin 30.0
Cetyl alcohol 1.0
b Distilled water 44.2
Borax 0.8
c Colour one microspatula-full
d Perfume one to three drops

Method: Disperse the colour base in the melted fats (these should be heated to 70°C). Add the aqueous phase at the same temperature. Mix and stir well. Add the perfume at 35°C.

4 *White Rouge*
Zinc oxide 40.0
Zinc stearate 10.0
White petroleum jelly 50.0
Perfume one drop
Preservative (Nipagin M) one microspatula-full

Method:
1 Mix and sieve the powder through fine muslin.
2 Warm and melt petroleum jelly in a beaker.
3 Add to the powder and mix thoroughly in a mortar and pestle.

5 *Cream Rouge for Greasy Skin*
Triethanolamine stearate 15.0
Glycerine 30.0
Distilled water 55.0
Preservative (Nipagin M) one microspatula-full
Colour one microspatula-full
Titanium dioxide one microspatula-full

Method: Warm the triethanolamine stearate with water (65°C). Stir until cool (35°C). Add the glycerine and colours, which have been thoroughly mixed.

6 *Dry Skin Rouge*
Triethanolamine stearate 15.0
Petroleum jelly 15.0
Glycerine 7.0
Lanolin 10.0
Distilled water 53.0
Preservative (Nipagin M) one microspatula-full

Method: Melt the petroleum jelly, lanolin and glycerine to 60°–70°C. Add the triethanolamine stearate and preservative to the water and heat to the same temperature. Add this to the oil phase. Add the colour.

7   *Dry Rouge*

Kaolin	16.0
Zinc oxide	16.0
Magnesium stearate	2.0
Zinc stearate	1.0
Magnesium carbonate	3.0
Talc (extra fine)	62.0
Colour	one microspatula-full
Perfume	one drop
Preservative (Nipagin M)	one microspatula-full

Method: Add the perfume to the magnesium carbonate, cover and allow to stand for half an hour. Mix the remaining powders thoroughly and sieve through fine muslin. Add the magnesium carbonate and then the required colours.

Appendix I
Further reading

BOOKS
Complete Herbal, N. Culpeper, Foulsham (1972).
**Cosmetic Science,* Ed. A. W. Middleton, Butterworth (1959).
Cosmetics, E. Sagarin, Interscience (1972).
Handbook of Cosmetic Science, H. W. Hibbott, Pergamon (1963).
Modern Cosmeticology, R. G. Harry, Leonard Hill (to be published 1973).
**Natural Beauty Secrets,* Deborah Rutledge, Arlington Books (1969).
Perfumes, Cosmetics and Soaps, W. A. Poucher, Chapman & Hall (1959).
**Technique of Beauty Products,* Leonard Hill.
**The Practice of Modern Perfumery,* P. Jellinek, Leonard Hill (1954).

Booklets
New Beauty, C. Perry, Cosmetic (Ealing) Co. Ltd.
Cosmetic Science, J. Gostelow, Shell Educational Services (available free to teachers).

Journals
Manufacturing Chemist, Morgan-Grampian, monthly.
Soap, Perfumery and Cosmetics, United Trade Press, monthly.

Also available: Griffin Technical Studies Kit, Cosmetic Science. (See Appendix IV for address.)

*Out of print, but will probably be available in your library.

Appendix II
Raw materials

The manufacturers listed below are those that the author can recommend. However, some of the materials are available from several manufacturers.

Name	Composition
*Abracol GMS	Water dispersible glyceryl monostearate
*Abracol GSP	Modified glyceryl monostearate (self-emulsifying)
*Abracol LDS	Based on a fatty alcohol ethylene oxide condensate and a polyhydric alcohol fatty acid ester
*Abracol PGS	Cream coloured wax. M.P. 46°C. Self-emulsifying form of propylene glycol monostearate
*Abracol SPS	Glyceryl monostearate, based on modified polyoxethylene fatty acid derivative. Fairly soft cream coloured wax. M.P. 45°C
*Abracol VPX	Absorption base of wool wax alcohol type

Notes: *Non-ionic emulsifying agents

Glyceryl monostearate is a useful stabilizer for oil in water and water in oil emulsions. Most glyceryl monostearates commercially available include added coap and sulphated fatty alcohol

Acacia	Obtained from *Acacia senegal* and other species. Occur in round or ovoid colourless to pale yellow lumps, soluble in water
Acetone	Colourless clear volatile highly inflammable liquid
Acetoglycerides	Vary from pale yellow to water white liquids and waxes (M.P. 30°–32°C)

Uses	Manufacturer (see Appendix III for addresses)
Used as an emulsifying agent in oil and water emulsions	Bush, Boake, Allen Ltd Evans Medical British Drug Houses
Oil in water emulsifying agent for cosmetic cream	As above
Oil in water emulsifying agent for firm cosmetic creams. Used mainly in cold wave cream	As above
Used in water in oil emulsions with triethanolamine soaps	As above
Used in the preparation of hair creams and nourishing creams (water in oil emulsions)	As above
Used in cosmetic creams	As above
Oil in water emulsifying agent, thickening agent, emollient agent	British Drug Houses Evans Medical
Used in nail varnish and nail varnish remover	Evans Medical
Modifying and blending agent for waxes and oils in lipsticks, improves the thixotropic properties, makes the lipstick firm and makes for easier application	Bush, Boake, Allen Ltd

Name	Composition
Acetoglyceride L/C	Mixed esters of glycerol (triglyceride) derived from blend of fatty acids. Pale amber liquid
Acetoglyceride S/C	Similar in composition to above but based on stearic acid. It is a solid wax
Aeromatt	Cosmetic precipitated calcium carbonate
Agar	Dried gelatinous substance obtained from seaweeds
Algin	Sodium alginate
Alginates	Colloidal substances manufactured from kelp
Almond Oil	Fixed oil from the seeds of prumas. Occurs as a pale yellow oil insoluble in water. Slightly soluble in alcohol. Fatty acids of almond oil, saturated: myristic, palmitic; unsaturated: oleic
Alum (or Potassium Aluminium Sulphate)	Crystalline double sulphate of either potassium or ammonia aluminium sulphate
Aluminium Chloride	Occurs in white or slightly yellowish crystals which are deliquescent or a white or yellowish powder
Aluminium Stearates (Higel No. 1, Nogel No. 2)	These vary in composition between aluminium hydroxy-distearate and aluminium hydroxide. They are covalent, being derived from a weak acid and a weak base
Ammonia Solution	10% solution or even more dilute
Amyl Acetate	Colourless neutral liquid prepared by esterifying amyl alcohol with glacial acetic acid

APPENDIX II

Uses	Manufacturer
Used in emulsions and lotions, gives added richness to fatty skin creams and also greater emolliency	Bush, Boake, Allen
Gives more body to emulsions	As above
Used in high grade face powders	John & E. Sturge Ltd
Used in preparation of certain glycerine jellies for use on chapped hands	
Used as a stabilizer in emulsions and thickening agent	Alginate Industries
Stabilizers and thickening agents	As above
Used in skin foods as an emollient and also in anti-wrinkle creams	Evans Medical
Used in astringent lotions, skin foods, after shave lotions	Bush, Boake, Allen Ltd British Drug Houses
Very effective deodorant. It is the aluminium which reacts with and precipitates the skin proteins, with the consequential obstruction of the sweat pores	As above
Used to make gels	As above
Used in hair dyes, permanent wave solutions, in some emulsions and as water softeners; also in insect bite preparations	British Drug Houses Evans Medical Hopkinson
Used in the manufacture of nail varnish	Bush, Boake, Allen Ltd British Drug Houses Evans Medical

Name	Composition
Aniseed oil	Volatile oil distilled from dried raw fruits of star-anise. Occurs in pale yellow liquid
Antiviray W.S	Pale coloured liquid, oil-soluble sunscreening agent. Specific gravity 1.061
Arachis Oil (Synonyms: Ground Nut Oil, Peanut Oil)	Pale yellow liquid, slightly soluble in alcohol. *Fatty acids.* Saturated: myristitic, palmitic, stearic, arachidic; behenic, unsaturated: oleic, linoleic
Arlacels (Span & Tween) (*Registered Trade Marks*)	
Arlacel 20	Sorbitan monolaurate, yellow oily liquid
Arlacel 40	Sorbitan monopalmitate, cream coloured wax
Arlacel 60	Sorbitan monostearate, light coloured cream, waxy solid
Arlacel 80	Sorbitan monoleate, yellow oily liquid
Arlacel 83	Light yellow oily liquid insoluble in water
Avocado Pear Oil	Obtained from fleshy parts of avocado pear, green oil or bleached. Slightly cloudy oil, contains most vitamins
Baker's Yeast	BPC (compressed distillers' yeast). Contains invertase, maltase, ergosterol, zymosterol, glycogen, Vit B_1 and B_2
Beeswax	Complicated mixture of hydrocarbon alcohols occuring as esters
Bentonite (Devon Clay)	Colloidal clay derived from volcanish aluminium silicate. Creamy to greyish coloured coloured powder, possesses very great adsorptive properties
Benzoic Acid	C_6H_5COOH
Benzoin (tincture of)	Contains free and combined benzoic acid and cinnamic acid up to 38%, together with vanillin benzoresinol, styrol, stryoracin and ethereal oil, and balsamic resin

Uses

Used for flavouring toothpaste

Used in the preparation of anti-sunburn creams, lotions, oils and aerosol sprays

Used as a substitute for almond oil or olive oil in cosmetic creams, skin foods, brilliantines

The Arlacels are used as emulsifying agents in water, in oil and water creams, in cold creams and in all-purpose creams

Used as a lubricant, and can reduce the surface tension of liquids

Used in face masks

Employed as an emulsifying agent with borax stabilizer in lipsticks and hair creams

Used as a thickening agent in face cream, liquid powder, face masks (used to absorb greasiness). Gelling agent. Oil in water emulsifier. Stabilizer for water in oil emulsifier

Preservative

Tincture used as a stimulant and antiseptic. Can be used in face lotions for irritable condition of the skin

Manufacturer

Osborne Garrett & Co

Bush, Boake, Allen Ltd

Evans Medical

Atlas Company (English Agents: Honeywell & Stein Ltd)

P. Samuelson & Co

Any baker's shop or
Evans Medical

Pothe Hill & Co

Evans Medical

As above

Name	Composition
Bergamot Oil	Contains 36–45% linalyl acetate. Volatile oil expressed from rind of the fresh fruit, *Citrus bergamia*. Yellow, green or brownish yellow liquid
Biosulphur Powder	Consists of very finely divided and highly active sulphur. It also contains stabilizing, protective colloids which retard the deposition of the sulphur in suspensions. Yellowish, very fine powder
Borax	Sodium borate—sodium tetraborate or pyro borax. Occurs in form of transparent colourless crystals. Can be obtained by boiling calcium borates with sodium carbonate solution
Boric Acid	Occurs as colourless crystals or powder
Bromo Acids	Two substances—dibromo and tetrabromo fluoresceins. Dibromo—orange powder. Tetrabromo—pink powder
Butyl Stearate	Mixture of butyl stearate and butyl palmitate. Colourless liquid
Calcium Carbonate	$CaCO_3$ Precipitated chalk. White odourless powder (various densities and grades)
Calcium Phosphate (dibasic)	White crystalline powder
Calcium Stearate	$(C_{17}H_{35}COO)_2Ca$
Calendula (Marigold) Oil	Reddish yellow oil. Blossoms are processed and extracted with a vegetable oil. Contains a lipid. Soluble constituent of the calendula blossom

APPENDIX II

Uses	Manufacturer
Eau de Cologne toilet water, hair oils and creams—has the property of assisting to form skin tan	Osborne Garrett & Co Bush, Boake, Allen Ltd
Used for the treatment of greasy skins (using creams, masks and powders). Also used for combating dandruff, (creams and shampoos)	Bio Cosmetics
Mild detergent properties. Antiseptic. Used as an emulsifier in conjunction with beeswax for cold creams, vanishing creams	British Drug Houses Hopkinson & Williams
Used in talcum powders, baby powders, cold creams, in a beeswax borax emulsion	British Drug Houses Hopkinson & Williams
These impart orange or reddish stain to lipsticks	Williams of Hounslow
Used as a water repelling plasticiser in nail varnish and nail varnish remover. Sometimes used in lipsticks and in the oil phase of a cleansing cream	Bush, Boake, Allen Ltd Evans Medical British Drug Houses
Used in talcs, face powders, baby powders	British Drug Houses Evans Medical John & E. Sturge Ltd Marchon Products
Abrasive in toothpastes	As above
Water in oil emulsifying agent	As above
Used for dry, cracked and chapped skin (in emulsions for this purpose)	Bio Cosmetics

Name	Composition
Camphor	White crystalline substance obtained from cinnamon camphors
Candelilla Wax	Obtained from *Candelilla* weed. Colour varies from pale grey to dark grey to brown. M.P. 67–68°C
Carbitol	Diethylene glycol monoethyl ether. $C_5H_{12}O_3$. Colourless liquid, faint odour. Miscible with glycerine, alcohol and water
Carbon Black (Cosmetic black)	Carbon. Can be obtained in three shades. Masstone, 10% dispersion in TiO_2, 2% dispersion in TiO_2
Carnauba Wax	Hard wax complex mixture of higher fatty alcohol esters. Yellow or brown or white gold
Carragheen	Dried seaweed
Carrot Oil CLR	Deep red fatty oil, odourless. Soluble in oils and fats
Casein	Nitrogenous constituent of milk (phosphoprotein)
Castile Soap (see Dental Soap)	
Castor Oil (Oleum Ricini)	Colourless or pale yellow viscous liquid. Fatty acid of castor oil consisting of 98% unsaturated acid, 86% ricinoleic, $8\frac{1}{2}$% oleic and $3\frac{1}{2}$% linoleic, together with 3% saturated acid
Caustic Soda (see Sodium Hydroxide)	
Ceresine Wax	A refined form of ozokerite obtained in white or yellow pieces. M.P. 60°–80°C
Cetrimide	Cetylrime thylammonium bromide
Cetyl Alcohol (Synonym: Palmityl Alcohol)	$C_{16}H_{33}OH$ Obtained as slab or cube or waxy scaly powder. M.P. 48°–49°C

Uses	Manufacturer
Used as an antiseptic	Bio Cosmetics
Used in lipstick formulae	Pothe Hill & Co
Can be used as an humectant in place of glycerine, in vanishing creams, hand creams, hand lotions and shaving creams	Honeywell Atlas Co
Used in eye-liner and mascara	Williams of Hounslow
Used in creams (furniture and cosmetic) and lipsticks to give a firmer preparation	As above
Mucilaginous extract used as an emulsifying agent, stabilizer and thickening agent	Bio Cosmetics
Used in emulsion and conditioning creams	As above
Used as a constituent for massage creams. Thickening agent and oil in water emulsifying agent	British Drug Houses
Used in lipsticks, brilliantines, nail varnish as a plasticiser and in nail polish remover	Evans Medical
Used in cosmetic cream to give a firmer produced lipstick, etc., and to prevent separation of the oils	Pothe Hill & Co Croda Limited
Used as an antiseptic and oil in water emulsifying agent	Evans Medical British Drug Houses
It is a stabilizer for oil in water emulsion. Emollient and weaker water in oil emulsifying agent. Can be incorporated in lipsticks, powders and rouges	Pothe Hill & Co British Drug Houses Evans Medical

Name	Composition
Chlorohexide	White crystals, soluble in water, with alkaline reaction
Cholesterol	Sterol contained in wool alcohols and in animal nerve tissue and egg yolk
Cinnamon (Oil of)	Volatile oil distilled from *Cinnamon cassia*. Contains 80% cinnamic aldehyde. Yellowish liquid
Citric Acid	Found in fruits (citrus), pears, lemons, limes. Colourless translucent crystals or white powder
Citrol 4ML 10ML 4MS 10MS 4MR 10MR 4MO 10MO	Polyglycol 400 monolaurate ,, 1000 ,, ,, 400 monostearate ,, 1000 ,, ,, 400 monoriconolide ,, 1000 ,, ,, 400 monoleum ,, 1000 monoleum
Cithrol No. 6	MS mono ester of polyethylene glycol 1000 and stearic acid
Civet Infusion	Obtained from civet cat. (Musky substance)
Clove Oil	Contains 82–90% Eugenol, small quantities of vanillin and methylamylketone furfural. Colourless to pale yellow liquid
Cocoa Butter	Oleum theo broma, consisting of glycerine, stearic palmites, oleic and arachidic and linoleic acid
Coconut Oil	Copra oil
Collone AC	Fatty alcohol ethylene oxide. Condensation product. Non-ionic
Collone HV	Emulsifying wax based on cetyl alcohol
Collone SE & SEC	Emulsifying wax BP. Saturated fatty alcohol containing a proportion of sulphated alcohol

Uses	Manufacturer
Used as an antiseptic	I.C.I.
Used in skin foods, muscle oils, water in oil emulsifier	Bio Cosmetics British Drug Houses
Used in toothpastes	Evans Medical
Used in rinses, bath salts, nail bleaches, astringent lotions	British Drug Houses
Used in cosmetic emulsions	Croda Limited
Used in cosmetic emulsions	
Used in perfumes. (Artificial substance is now used)	P. Samuelson & Co
Used in perfumes as a flavouring agent	Bush, Boake, Allen Ltd P. Samuelson & Co
Used in lipstick formulae and in cosmetic creams as an emollient	British Drug Houses Evans Medical Hopkinson & Williams
Used in shampoos	As above
Oil in water emulsifying agent, gives a fluid emulsion. M.P. 27°C	Glovers Chemicals
Oil in water emulsifying agent. M.P. 75°C	As above
Oil in water emulsifying agent. M.P. 75°C	As above

Name	Composition
Collone QAC	Cetrimide emulsifying wax BPC. Contains higher saturated fatty alcohols, having incorporated a proportion of a quaternary ammonium compound
Colours (See Appendix III)	
Colours	—
Colours	—
Copper Chloride	$CuCl_2$
Copper Sulphate	$CuSO_4$
Crill K1, 3, 16 Sorbitan Monolaurate	Oil soluble non-ionic surface active agent. pale clear amber coloured viscous liquid, Soluble in mineral oils, alcohol. It is dispersible in water, alkali and acids
Crillet 4	Polyoxethylene derivative of sorbitan monooleate. Pale yellow liquid soluble in water and alcohol
Crill 5, 6	Polyoxethylene derivative of sorbital monostearate
Crodamol DA Crodamol ML	These are speciality esters, odourless, tasteless, soluble in hydro-alcoholic-based preparations. *Crodamol DA*—Di-isopropyl adipate, White liquid. *Crodamol ML*—Myristyl lactate, White yellow soft solid
Curd Soap	Mainly sodium stearate

Uses	Manufacturer
Used in emulsions which are absorbed into the skin or hair more easily	Glovers Chemicals
For powders, lipstick, eye shadow and bath salts	Bush, Boake, Allen Ltd Williams of Hounslow D. F. Anstead
For shampoo	Osborne Garrett & Co
For creams and lotions, rouges and hair dyes	Bush, Boake, Allen Ltd Williams of Hounslow Osborne, Garrett & Co
Used in hair dyes (copper dyes)	Hopkinson, Williams of Hounslow
Used in hair dyes (copper dyes)	Williams of Hounslow
Wetting agent. Spreading and foaming agent used in hair dressing and hair waving preparations	Croda Limited
Used in conjunction with Crill 4 for oil in water emulsion	As above
Used with Crill K3 for oil in water emulsions	As above
Used as emollients and in bath oils	As above
Oil in water emulsifying agent	Evans Medical

Name	Composition
Dastar	Cholesterol (50%) obtained from wool wax
Dental Soap Powder	White or creamy, neutral and tasteless
Dichlorophene	White powder
Dicalcium Phosphate (see Calcium phosphate, dibasic)	
Diglycol Laurates	Diethylene glycol monolaurate
Diglycol Stearate S	Crodamat
Dihydroxy Acetone	Formed together with a little glyceraldehyde where glycerine is oxidized with nitric acid. White crystalline solid. M.P. 69–72°C
Diethylene Glycol Monostearate	Water dispersible wax $C_{17}H_{35}COOC_2H_4OC_2H_9O_{11}$
Di-isopropanola-mine	$(CH_3CHOHCH_2)_2NH$
Dimethyl Phthalate (Palatinol M)	Colourless, odourless liquid
Empicol ESB 30	Sodium lauryl ether sulphate (liquid)
Empicol LM	Sodium lauryl sulphate (powder)
Empicol LQ	Monoethanolamine salts of sulphated lauryl alcohol (liquid)
Empicol LZ	Various grades of sodium lauryl sulphate (powder)
Empicol TCR, TC34	Triethanolamine ammonium lauryl sulphate (liquid)
Empicol TL (HO)	Triethanolamine salts of sulphated lauryl alcohol (liquid)
Empilan BQ AO AP	Polyethylene glycol esters of fatty acids

APPENDIX II 141

Uses	Manufacturer
Water in oil emulsifying agent	Croda Limited
Used in toothpaste	
Used in creams, powders and other preparations as an antiseptic	Evans Medical British Drug Houses
Emulsifier for fluid emulsions and lotions (cleansing milks, hand lotions)	Rex Campell & Co
Used as an emulsifier for oils, fats, waxes where a stable neutral viscous cream is required. Pearly vanishing creams, night creams, etc	As above
Used as a self-tanning agent in conjunction with Antiviray sun screening agent	Bush, Boake, Allen Rex Campbell
Used as an oil in water emulsifying agent	Rex Campbell & Co
Used in after-shave lotions	Osborne Garrett Evans Medical
Used in insect repellent lotions	Bush, Boake, Allen Ltd
Wetting agent giving stable foams for use in shampoos	Marchon Products
Detergent used in shampoos	As above
Detergent used in shampoos	As above
Emulsifying, wetting and foaming agent	As above
Detergent and ingredients of shampoos	As above
Detergent used in shampoos	As above
Wetting agents	As above

Name	Composition
Empilan CDE	Dialkylolamides of various fatty acids. Liquid paste, golden yellow
Empilan CME	Fatty acids alkylolamides CME monoethanolamide. Waxy flakes, cream colour, dispersible in hot water. Stable to acids and alkalis under certain conditions
Empilan GMS (Non-self-emulsifying grade)	Glycerine monostearates. White wax-like powders. Contain fatty acid and glycerine. M.P. 55°–61°C
Empilan LDE	Dialkyloamide of various fatty acids (lauric fatty acid). Ratio: 1 diamolamine to 1 fatty acid
Empilan SE (Self-emulsifying grade)	
Empilan S	Glycerine ethylene oxide and glycol condensation product
Empiwax SK	Self-emulsifying wax based on stearyl alcohol
Emulsene 1219	Fatty alcohol ethylene oxide condensate with a higher fatty alcohol
Emulsene 1220	Ethylene oxide derivative of a fatty alcohol with a high fatty alcohol
Eosin (Tetra bromo fluorescein)	Prepared by dissolving fluorescein in acetic acid and adding bromine. Eosin is precipitated as a pink powder, insoluble in water, soluble in alcohol
Estax No. 25	Triethanolamine stearate
Ethyl Alcohol (Ethanol)	Colourless mobile liquid miscible with water (known also as toilet spirit)

Uses	Manufacturer
Foam stabilizers and solubilizers in detergents (shampoos). Increases the total detergency	Marchon Products
Foam stabilizer and booster in liquid and powder detergent (e.g. shampoos)	As above
Weak emulsifying agents for oils, fats and waxes in creams. Have emollient properties	As above
Used as a foam stabilizer when used in conjunction with lauryl sulphate	As above
Non-ionic emulsifier	As above
Oil in water emulsifying agent	As above
Emulsifying agent for use in the presence of weak acids or electrolytes	Bush, Boake, Allen Ltd Evans Medical British Drug Houses
Emulsifying agent used in the preparation of thin lotions and emulsions	As above
Used to give indelibility to lipsticks	Williams of Hounslow
Oil in water emulsifier for cosmetic creams	
Used in making perfume, hair tonics, pre and after shave lotions, setting lotions. Concentration of alcoholic solutions greater than 50% precipitate skin proteins, assist in removing grease. In order to exhort a lubricant action, castor oils are added	

Name	Composition
Ethyl Butex (Nipagin A)	Ethyl p-hydroxybenzoate
Ethylene Glycol Monostearate	Self-emulsifying oil in water emulsifying agent. $C_{17}H_{65}COOC_2H_4OH$
Fat Stabilizer CLR	Antioxidant. Contains tocopherols
Flavours	—
Fluilan	Mixture of liquid esters of wool fat
Fluorescein (Eosin)	Obtained by heating resorcinol with phthalic anhydride. Dark brown powder
Fullers Earth	Variety of clay-like materials which absorb oil and grease. Chemical composition varies. Consists of hydrated silicates of magnesium, calcium and aluminium
Gelatin	Protein obtained from certain animal tissues such as ligaments, bones, etc
Glauber's Salt (see Sodium Sulphate)	
Glyceryl Monostearate (see also Empilan GMS)	Waxy substance, M.P. 57°C
Glycerine	$C_3H_8O_3$ Clear colourless hygroscopic liquid
Glycol Laurate Synonyms: Mono Empilan AP or Empicol A/Q100	Paste or solid soluble in water ⎫ Liquid soluble in water ⎭
Gum Tragacanth (Synonym: Goats Horn)	Mixture of tragacanthic acid and a neutral polysaccharide and small quantity of glycoside. Thin, flattened and translucent flakes, slightly soluble in water

Uses	Manufacturer
Preservative	Nipa Laboratories
Is a stabilizer (if pure) for oil in water emulsions and gives a pearly sheen to shampoos	Marchon Products
Retards rancidity of fats and fatty oils. Basic material for emulsified and oily cosmetics	Bio Cosmetics Ltd
For lipsticks	Bush, Boake, Allen Ltd International Flavours
Water in oil emulsifying agent	Croda Limited
Used as a staining agent in lipsticks	Williams of Hounslow
Used in powders and face masks	Evans Medical
This is a stabilizer for oil in water emulsions and thickening agent. Can be used with gum tragacanth to increase viscosity of emulsion	
Used in cosmetic creams such as vanishing creams	Rex Campell & Co
Used in all preparations. Improves the spreading properties of creams. It acts as a humectant. Used in after shave creams, all purpose creams, cleansing creams, vanishing creams, etc	British Drug Houses Evans Medical
Emulsifier and wetting agent	Rex Campbell & Co
Used as a fixative in hair creams, creams and setting lotions. Suspending agent for liquid powders, toothpaste and hand creams	British Drug Houses Evans Medical

Name	Composition
Hartolan	Wool alcohols
Henna	Dried powdered leaves of *Lawsonia spinosa* and *Lawsonia inemus*. Removed from the plant before flowering. Active ingredient is Lawsone
Honey	Chiefly dextrose and laevulose, with a *little* glucose, wax and volatile oil
Hydrogen Peroxide 5 vols	Prepared by the action of a dilute acid upon the metallic peroxide. H_2O_2. Colourless liquid
Hygroplex HHG	Contains mono and disaccharides in natural combinations with amino acids, together with carbamide.
Hydroxystearin Sulphate	Sulphated hydrogenated castor oil
Irish Moss	Carragheen dried seaweed
Isopropyl Alcohol	Colourless liquid, slight odour
Isopropyl Lineolate	Ester prepared from essential fatty acid (sometimes referred to as Vitamin F). Consists of linoleic, linolemic and arachidonic unsaturated fatty acids. Pale yellow liquid, slight fatty odour
Isopropyl Myristate	Colourless odourless liquid. It is a mixture of myristate and small amounts of other esters. High boiling point and low volatility
Isopropyl Palmitate	Similar to the myristate but contains the ester of palmitic acid. It is a solid. Excellent solvent
Isopropyl Palmitate Stearate	Contains saturated fatty acids

APPENDIX II

Uses	Manufacturer
Water in oil emulsifying agent	Croda Limited
Used as a hair dye or hair brightening rinse. The content of Lawsone makes it a substantive dye for keratin in acid solutions	Evans Medical
Used in small proportion, gives a smooth feel to skin. Used also in massage cream	As above Any shop
Used as a bleaching agent in cosmetic creams and for bleaching hair. With creams it needs a stabilizer or preservative	British Drug Houses
Used as a moisturizing agent in dry skin creams	Bio Cosmetics
Oil in water emulsifying agent	
Aqueous extract used as an emollient and thickener for hand creams	Any Health Store Bio Cosmetics Ltd
Used as a substitute for ethyl alcohol in hair tonics, colognes, perfumes	Evans Medical Bush, Boake, Allen Ltd British Drug Houses
Used as an emollient. Has healing properties in skin conditioning creams	Bush, Boake, Allen
Used in all types of cosmetics, lotions, creams, lipsticks, and as a partial replacement of vegetable and mineral oils	Evans Medical Bush, Boake, Allen Ltd British Drug Houses
Emollient and lubricant, used in skin foods. Has no harmful effect on the skin	As above
Used in emulsions and lotions as softening and lubricating agent	Bush, Boake, Allen

Name	Composition
Japan Wax	Hard wax-like fat consisting mainly of glycerides of palmitic and similar fatty acids
Kaolin (hydrated aluminium silicate)	China clay, porcelain clay. It is a hydrated aluminium silicate, white or yellowish white powder
Kerosene (see Mineral Oil)	
Lactic Acid	Colourless liquid, slight odour, miscible with water
Lambutol Wax (Lambutol N2)	Mixture of fatty alcohols with polyethylene glycol ester of fatty alcohols
Lanette Wax	Cetyl/stearyl alcohol mixture
Lanette Wax SX	Partially sulphated cetyl/stearyl alcohol mixture. M.P. 50°C. Appearance—wax-like, varies from white to yellow
Lanolin (wool wax) (anhydrous lanolin, anhydrous wool fat)	Composed of 94% esters, which on hydrolysis yield a mixture of complex alcohols and fatty acids. It is the purified anhydrous fat-like substance from wool of sheep
Liquid Lanolin (see Fluilan)	
Laurex 18	Stearyl alcohol
CS	Cetostearyl alcohol
Lecithin	Ovolecithin (egg lecithin) phospholutein essential constituent of animal and vegetable cells, soya bean (animal nerve tissue), white waxy substance insoluble in water
Lemon Oil	Volatile oil from fresh peel of lemon
Lime Water	0·15% calcium hydroxide solution. Clear, colourless liquid
Lithium Stearate	Lithium content 2.4 Free stearic acid content 0.25
Magnesium Carbonate (light: "levis", heavy: "pond")	$3MgCO_3 \cdot Mg(OH)_2 \cdot 3H_2O$

APPENDIX II

Uses	Manufacturer
Used as a hardening agent to give more firmness	Pothe Hill & Co
Used in talcum and baby powders, rouges, powder creams and face powders	Evans Medical
Used in astringent lotions	
Non-ionic wax for stabilizing oil in water emulsions	Ronsheim & Moore
Auxiliary emulsifier for cosmetic creams	As above
Self-emulsifying wax forming oil in water emulsions, used in cosmetic creams	As above
Used as an emollient in skin foods, hand creams, baby creams and in lipsticks. It is a stabilizer for a water in oil emulsion. It is used in creams for prevention of dermatitis	Evans Medical British Drug Houses
Hydrophobic stabilizer for oil in water emulsions	Marchon Products
Oil in water emulsifying agent with emollient and antioxidant properties, used in muscle and anti-wrinkle creams	
Used to give lemon odour to creams	
Used to aid emulsification in creams, lotions or emulsions made with almond oil	British Drug Houses Evans Medical
Used in baby powders, dusting powders. Can be used as an auxiliary filler for paste. Emulsifying agent	Bush, Boake, Allen British Drug Houses
Used to incorporate perfume for face powder, talcum and baby powders	John & E. Sturge Ltd

Name	Composition
Magnesium Hydroxide	Prepared by boiling light magnesium oxide with excess of water, draining and drying in thin layers at a temperature not greater than 100°C. White amorphous powder, insoluble in water
Magnesium Stearate	Fine white bulky powder compound of magnesium and stearic acid
Magnesium Sulphate (Epsom Salts)	$MgSO_4\ 7H_2O$
Manucol	Sodium alginate
Manutex (Manutex AKP)	Sodium alginate
Menthol	Secondary alcohol obtained from peppermint oil or prepared synthetically by hydrogenation of thyme. It occurs as colourless crystals, soluble in alcohol
Mineral Oil or White Oil (Special for cosmetic purposes)	These include the kerosene, technical white oils and medicinal paraffins
Montan Wax	Crude wax extracted from brown coal by benzene or benzol. Pure montan wax has as its main constituent "Montanic Acid" $C_{27}H_{52}COOH$, in association with unsaturated hydrocarbons
Morpon GH	Cetrimide
Musk	This comes from a small gland situated near the sexual organs of the male musk deer and musk rat
Nipagin A	Ethyl p. hydroxybenzoate
Nipagin M	Methyl p.hydroxybenzoate
Nipantiox IF	Butylated hydroxyanisoll
Nipasol M	Propyl p.hydroxybenzoate
Novol (see Oleyl Alcohol)	

Uses

Used in milk of magnesia pastes and creams, to cure "acid" skin

Used in face powders, baby powders and foot powders

Used in reducing bath salts

Thickening and stabilizing agent, gel formation

Thickening and stabilizing agent

Used in insect bite preparations, pre-shave lotions and brushless shaving creams

Used as emollient and skin lubricant

Used to give hardness to stick cosmetics

Antiseptic and detergent

Used as a fixative in perfumes

Preservative

Preservative

Antioxidant for oils and fats

Preservative

Manufacturer

Evans Medical

As above
British Drug Houses

British Drug Houses
Evans Medical

Alginate Industries

As above

Evans Medical

Osborne Garrett Ltd
Evans Medical

Pothe Hill

Glovers Chemicals

Bush, Boake, Allen Ltd

As above

As above

As above

As above

Name	Composition
Oleic acid	Occurs as colourless or yellowish oily liquid obtained by hydrolyses of fats which contain glycerides of oleic acid
Oleyl Alcohol or Oleic Alcohol	Occurs in head and blubber oils of sperm whales. Clear yellow liquid
Olive Oil	Oleum olivae glyceryl ester of certain fatty acids. *Composition:* Saturated: myristic, palmitic, stearic and arachidic acid. Unsaturated: oleic and linoleic. A pale yellow liquid, soluble in 90% alcohol
Orange Flower Water	Distillation of orange flower petals and alcohol
Ozokerite	Natural occurring wax found in the vicinity of petroleum springs. Occurs in dark brown, yellow or white hard wax. Pure white used in cosmetic formulations
Palatinol M (see Dimethyl Phthalate)	
Palmityl Alcohol (see Cetyl Alcohol)	
Palm Kernel Oil	Contains capric, caprylic, palmitic and stearic saturated acid. Unsaturated: oleic acid. A yellowish, fatty substance
Paraffin Wax (hard)	Mixture of solid hydrocarbons
Peanut Oil (see Arachis Oil)	
Pectin	Carbohydrate substance obtained from citrus fruits, apples and pears and in plants
Peppermint Oil	Oil distilled from fresh flowers, i.e. tops of mentha piperita, and rectified. Colourless, pale yellow or green/yellow liquid
Perfumes	(see appendix III)

APPENDIX III 153

Uses	Manufacturer
Used in permanent waving solution, cold and vanishing creams	British Drug Houses Evans Medical
Superfattening agent in emulsions, creams, lotions, lipsticks, as a dispersing agent for eosins	Bush, Boake, Allen Ltd Evans Medical
Used as an emollient in hair conditioning oils and creams	
Used in toilet water, perfumes and emulsions	Evans Medical
Used in lipsticks to give firmer stick	Pothe Hill & Co
Used in soaps and cleansing creams	Evans Medical
Used in mascara, cream rouges, liquefying cleansing creams	Pothe Hill & Co
Thickening agent	Evans Medical
Flavouring of toothpastes	Osborne Garrett Ltd
For creams, lotions, deodorants, lipsticks, bath salts, powders, shampoos, and nail preparations	Bush, Boake, Allen Ltd International Fragrances and Flavours Proprietory Perfumes P. Samuelson & Co. Norda Schimmel

Name	Composition
Perfumes	—
Petitgrain Oil	Distilled from the leaves and twigs of the bitter orange tree of Paraguay. Contains linalyl acetate and linalol
Petroleum Jelly (Soft Paraffin Molle)	Mixture of semi-solid hydrocarbons. Colour—yellow or *white*, which is mostly used in cosmetics
Phenoxetol	Ethylene glycol phenylether
Polowax	Cetylstearyl mixture
Polychol 5 (10152040)	Polyoxyethylene condensation product of wool wax alcohols. The degree of ethyoxylation increases with the number
Polyethylene Glycol 100 Stearate	—
Polyethylene Glycol 400 Monostearate (see Empilan BQ)	
Polyethylene Glycol 600 Monostearate. Crexa series	
Potassium Aluminium Sulphate (see Alum)	
Potassium Hydroxide	KOH. Caustic potash
Precipitated Chalk $CaCO_3$ (see Calcium Carbonate, precipitated)	
Precipitated Sulphur (Calcareous)	Prepared by precipitating sodium thiosulphate. A colloidal solution of sulphur is then obtained which gradually coagulates and gives a yellow precipitate
Progallin EA	Lauryl gallate

Uses	Manufacturer
For greasepaint and rouges	Bush, Boake, Allen Ltd British Drug Houses
Used in perfumes	Osborne Garrett
Creams, rouges, lipsticks, foundation creams, etc	Evans Medical British Drug Houses
Antiseptic or preservative	Nipa Laboratories
Oil in water emulsifying wax	Croda Limited
Emulsifying and emollient agent	
Stabilizer and it acts as an emollient in shaving creams	As above
Oil in water emulsifier for creams, shampoos and cold waving creams	Rex Campbell & Co
Used in the manufacture of soaps with fatty acids. Forms an emulsifier for vanishing creams	Evans Medical
Used in skin creams for acne and seborrhoeic dermatitis	As above
Antioxidant for preventing rancidity in emulsions	Nipa Laboratories

Name	Composition
Propylene glycol	$CH_3CHOHCH_2OH$
Pyrogallic Acid	Derived from gallic acid $C_6H_3(OH)_3$
Rose Water	Distillation of rose flower petals and alcohol
Saccharine (solution)	Sodium derivative of a benzoic sulphinide. White crystalline powder, odourless, soluble in water
Salycylic Acid	Occurs naturally as a methyl ester in oil of wintergreen. Colourless, odourless crystalline solid
Satinex	Fine talc
Sesame Oil	Fixed express oil of seeds of sesame
Silver Nitrate	$AgNO_3$, compound, solid. Made by the action of nitric acid on metallic silver. Soluble in water
Silicone (MS/200/10) (Dimethyl Silicone)	Colourless fluid
Sodium Alginate (Algin)	Manucol. Hydrophilic colloidal substances manufactured from kelp. Obtained as a white powder, soluble in water
Sodium Benzoate	C_5H_5COONa. Obtained by neutralizing benzoic acid with sodium carbonate
Sodium Bicarbonate (Bicarbonate of Soda)	$NaHCO_3$
Sodium Carbonate Anhydrous	Na_2CO_3

APPENDIX II 157

Uses	Manufacturer
Humectant in creams. Solvent for perfumes. Replaces glycerine. Preservative	Alginate Industries
Used in hair dyes	Evans Medical
Used in perfumes and emulsions	As above
Used for sweetening toothpastes	As above
Used as an antiseptic	As above
Used to give "slip" in powders	Bush, Boake, Allen Ltd Bio Cosmetics Ltd
Can be used instead of olive oil in creams	
Used in dyeing hair—a variety of shades e.g. from ash blond to brown. Tints obtained by increasing proportion of silver present in liquid	Evans Medical British Drug Houses Hopkinson & Co.
Used in emulsions as a stabilizer, particularly for barrier creams	Evans Medical
Used in hand jellies, face lotion and hand creams	Alginate Industries
Preservative in toothpaste and vanishing creams	British Drug Houses
Tooth powders and bath powders	As above
May be used in conjunction with fatty acids and then forms an emulsifier in creams. Used in soap powders and in bath salts	Evans Medical

Name	Composition
Sodium Carbonate Decahydrate (Washing Soda)	$Na_3CO.10H_2O$
Sodium Carbonate Monohydrate	$Na_2CO_3H_2O$. Odourless crystalling powder
Sodium Cetyl Sulphate	Powder, liquid or paste
Sodium Hydroxide (Caustic Soda)	NaOH
Sodium Hydroxybenzoate	Derivative of benzoic acid
Sodium Lauryl ether sulphate (see Empicol ESB 30)	
Sodium Lauryl Sulphate paste	$C_{12}H_{25}OSO_3Na$
Sodium Monolaurate	White power
Sodium Oleate	$C_{17}H_{33}COON$
Sodium Perborate	$NaBO_34H_2O$. White crystalline powder
Sodium Propanedioate (Synonym: Sodium Malonate)	Prepared from malonic acid by interaction of monochloroacetic acid and sodium cyanide, followed by hydrolyses of cyanocetic acid. White crystaline powder, soluble in water
Sodium Sesquicarbonate	$Na_2CO_3.NaHCO_3.2H_2O$
Sodium Silicate	Occurs as a white solid and solution
Sodium Sulphate (Glauber's Salt)	$Na_2SO_4.10H_2O$

APPENDIX II

Uses	Manufacturer
Used in bath salts	Evans Medical
Used in bath salts	As above
Used as emulsifier and wetting agent in shampoos	Bio Cosmetics
Used as an alkaline emulsifier in conjunction with fatty acid in vanishing creams	Evans Medical
Used as a preservative	Nipa Laboratories
Oil in water emulsifying agent	Bush, Boake, Allen Ltd British Drug Houses
Wetting and foaming agent in shampoos and emulsifying agent	Marchon Products
Solubilizer, detergent and emulsifying agent	Bush, Boake, Allen Ltd
Used in some hair rinses and shampoos (for blond hair), and in bath salts	Evans Medical
Used as an antiperspirant and in an emulsion of vanishing cream type	Evans Medical Bio Cosmetics
Stable and is easily coloured and perfumed, therefore used to make bath salts	As above
Used as a polishing agent in toothpaste and other emulsions	Marchon Products
Present in powdered sulphated preparations, used in shampoos	Bio Cosmetics Evans Medical

Name	Composition
Sodium Thiosulphate	Prepared by boiling a solution of sodium sulphate with sulphur for several hours. $Na_2S_2O_3$
Solan	Polyoxethylene lanolin derivative

Sorbitan Sesquioleate (see Arlacel 83)

Sorbitol	Occurs in cherries, plums, pears. Can be prepared from dextrose by treatment with hydrogen under pressure. Slightly soluble in methanol, ethanol, ascetic acid, phenol
Sorbitol Emulsifiers	
DO 33	Sorbitan di-oleate
MU 55	Polyoxetylene sorbitan mono-oleate

Soya Oil (see Vegetable Oils)

Span 20	Sorbitan monolaurate
Span 40	Sorbitan monopalmitate
Span 60	Sorbitan monostearate
Span 80	Sorbitan mono-oleate
Spermacetti	Solid wax consisting chiefly of cetyl palmitate
Spirit of Camphor	Camphor dissolved in alcohol
Stearyl Alcohol	Consists of over 95% octadecanol. Non toxic waxy compound. $C_{18}H_3OH$
Squalene (Acrylic Triterpenoid hydrocarbon $C_{30}H_{62}$	Composed of 90% liver oil of certain species of sharks
Starch	$(C_6H_{10}O_5)$ Polysaccharide obtained from wheat, rice, maize, potato
Stearic Acid	$C_{17}H_{35}COOH$. Occurs as a glyceride in tallow and other animal fats and oil and vegetable oil. White crystalline solid

APPENDIX II 161

Uses	Manufacturer
Used in hair dyes to develop or fix the colour	Evans Medical
Water soluble oil in water emulsifying agent	Croda Limited
Used as a humectant. Used in foundation creams. Can be used instead of glycerine. Retards evaporation and adds body to a cream	As above Rex Campell & Co
Water in oil emulsifying agent	As above
Oil in water emulsifying agent	As above
Stabilizer for oil in water emulsion	Honeywell & Stein Ltd
Stabilizer for oil in water emulsion	As above
Stabilizer for oil in water emulsion	As above
Stabilizer for oil in water emulsion	As above
Included in cold and other creams to improve gloss. Stabilizer for oil in water emulsions	Pothe Hill & Co
Used as an astringent	Evans Medical
Gives a firmer consistency to liquid emulsions. Produces a matt effect in oil/water emulsions	Bio Cosmetics
Used as an emollient and skin lubricant	As above
Used in face powders and baby powders. Thickening agent in cosmetic creams	
Used in vanishing creams and foundation creams and hair creams	Pothe Hill & Co

Name	Composition
Sulphated Castor Oil (Neutral)	(see Castor Oil)
Sulphated Castor Oil (Synonym: Turkey Red Oil)	Castor oil treated with concentrated sulphuric acid
Sulphonated "Lorol" DC	Sodium lauryl sulphate
Sulphonated "Lorol" TA	Triethanolamine lauryl sulphate
Sunflower Oil	(See Vegetable Oils)
Talc (French Chalk)	Hydrous silicate of magnesium $Mg_3Si_4O_{10}(OH)_2$. Occurs naturally
Tannic Acid	Ester-like compound of glucose
Tartaric Acid	COOH CH(OH) (CHOH) COOH. Main industrial source of tartaric acid is from argot, which is a brown crystalline deposit found on the sides of vessels when grape juice is fermented to make wine. Colourless crystalline solid, soluble in water, leaving a black residue—carbon
Teepol	Chiefly sodium higher alkyl sulphates
Terpineol (Synonym: Lilacia) $C_4H_{18}O$	Colourless viscous liquid, soluble in alcohol
Texafors *Type* A.B. C D.E. F. FN	Range of polyoxethylene derivative of type $RO(C_2H_4O)_nH$ R = Fatty alcohol R = Unsaturated fatty acid R = Glyceride oil R = Alkylphenic
Titanium Dioxide	TiO_2. White tasteless powder

APPENDIX II

Uses	Manufacturer
Oil in water emulsifying agent for cosmetic creams and lotions. Also used in soapless shampoos and as a wetting agent	Evans Medical
Detergent and wetting and emulsifying agent	Ronsheim & Moore Evans Medical
Detergent used in liquid soapless shampoos	As above
Used as an emollient	Bio Cosmetics Ltd
Used in face powders, foot powders and in baby powders	Evans Medical Bush, Boake, Allen Ltd
Used as an astringent in sunburn preventative creams	
Used in rinses for hair, and as an astringent	Evans Medical
Detergent, dispersing agent, emulsifying agent and used in soapless shampoos	Shell Chemicals
Is used as a constituent of perfumes for creams and soap	Osborne Garrett
Oil in water and water in oil emulsifying agents and stabilizers	Glovers Chemicals
Used in face powders for covering, also to make pale colours for lipsticks and powder creams	Bush, Boake, Allen Ltd Rex Campell & Co

Name	Composition
Toilet Spirit (see Ethyl Alcohol)	
Tragacanth (Goats Horn)	Gum obtained from *Astra galus*. Gummified mixture of tragacanth acid and a neutral poly saccharine
Triethanolamine	$(CH_2OH.CH_2)_3N$ Organic base. Colourless viscous alkaline liquid. Derivative of ammonia. Decomposes and darkens at high temperature
Triethanolamine TL(HO))	Ammonium Lauryl Sulphate (see Empicol
Triethanolamine Lauryl Sulphate (see Empicol TCR, TC34)	
Triethanolamine Stearate	Triethanolamine and stearic acid
Tween 20 40 60 65 80	Polyethylene sorbitan monolaurate Polyethylene sorbitan monopalmitate Polyethylene sorbitan monostearate Polyethylene sorbitan tri-stearate Polyethylene sorbitan mono-oleate
Vegetable Oil CLR (Synonym: Soya Oil)	Light yellow odourless selected soya oil. Low acid and peroxide number. Contains 0.2% lecithin. The oil is stabilized against rancidity. Soluble in oils, fats and lipid solvents
Vitamin F (Glyceric ester)	Complex compound of essential free fatty acids
Volpo Series VO N3 5 10 15 20	Odour-free polyoxethylene oleyl ethers. Soluble in alcohols. Glycols
Washing Soda (see Sodium Carbonate Decahydrate)	
Wheat Germ Oil (with Tocopherol)	Obtained by cold pressing fresh wheat germs. Suitable for vitamin E cosmetic treating preparations

Uses	Manufacturer
Thickening agent, stabilizer and oil in water emulsion fixative in hair creams	Evans Medical
Used for preparation of creams, cosmetic emulsions such as cleansing creams	Glovers Chemicals
Used as an emulsifier in the preparation of cleansing lotions and creams	Bush, Boake, Allen Ltd
Oil in water emulsifying agent	Honeywell & Stein Ltd
Oil in water emulsifying agent	As above
Oil in water emulsifying agent	As above
Oil in water emulsifying agent	As above
Oil in water emulsifying agent	As above
Basic material for emulsified and oily preparations	Bio Cosmetics
Counteracts dry and chapped skin as well as brittle and dull hair. Active substance for emulsified and oil skin and hair treating agents	As above
Used as emulsifiers for astringent creams and lotions. Dissolve bromo acids, act as spreading agents in bath oils and used for sunscreen gels and shampoos	Croda Limited
Used in emulsified and oily skin and hair preparations	Bio Cosmetics Ltd

Name	Composition
Witch Hazel Leaves (Hamamelis Winter Bloom)	Contains tannin gallic acid together with volatile oil. Dried leaves of hamamelis virginian, found in North America
Wool Alcohol	Prepared from wool fat. Contains about 30% lanosterol, 5 agnosterol and 40 inacibe alcohol
Zinc Oxide	ZnO (Synonym: Philosopher's Wool)
Zinc Stearate	Light, white amorphous powder. $Zn(C_{18}H_{35}O_2)_7$

Uses	Manufacturer
Used as an astringent in after shave lotion and in skin tonics	Evans Medical
Used to replace lanolins, as it has less odour than lanolin. Powerful water in oil emulsifying agent, emollient	As above
Imparts opacity to face powders	As above British Drug Houses
Used in face powders to give smoother powder	British Drug Houses

Appendix III
Perfumes and Colours

PERFUMES

Information supplied by
BUSH, BOAKE, ALLEN LTD.

Some perfumes for creams and lotions
Antholia 4996
Cologne SA1061
Gardenia 6031
Orange Flower P1700
Fougere 5532
Muguet 3544

Skin Tested
Citrus Bouquet
Amaryllis 5103
Lily of the Valley P2490
Parfume Cosmetique 5622
Bouquet 8A 1240

Perfumes for hand preparations
Apple Blossom 6564
Camomile PD0204
Rose 4547
Viburnum PD0663

Perfumes for foundation and liquid make-up
Cream foundation
Adelia 5479
Boutique Fragrance PD0638
Sari PD0642
Bouquet 5466
Parfume Cosmetique 5636

Liquid make-up
Esmerald 6414
Freesia 6325
Scilla 6355

(The skin tested perfumes can also be used.)

Perfumes for lipsticks
Lipstick perfume PD0363
Liparma 5515
Lipstick Perfume 6689
Boutique Fragrance PD0638

Perfumes for deodorants (stick)

Base Verte 6426
Esmeralda 6414
Lavender 6519
Fougere Amber 4402

Perfumes for antiperspirant creams and lotions

Coelia 4760
Illyria 6686
Lily of the Valley P2490

Perfumes for antiperspirant stick

Selva Verde 5172
Galanthus 4255

Perfumes for bath preparations

Dispersible bath oil
Carousel PD1005
Eau de Cologne PD0966
Boutique Chypre 6371

Bubble bath
Joanna 6574
Mimosa 5610
Spruce 6344

Perfumes for powders

Face powder
Coelia 6597
Cattleya 6507
Coeur d'or PD0156

Talcum powder
Honey Suckle 6189
Sandalwood 3708
Sycamore 4993
Bouquet Lemon PD0113
Amberwood 6696

Perfumes for hair preparations

Brilliantine
Valencia 6339
Carnation 1916
Fougere Amber 4402

Hair cream
 Cologne 1725
 Cologne Mandarinies 6318

Hair setting gell
 Citrus Bouquet 5177LS
 Herbal Cologne PDo283LS
 Magnolia P3052LS
 Spice PD0232LS

Shampoos
 Lemon Twist PD1040
 Motia 6566
 Savelia PD0935

Perfumes for sunscreen preparations

Sunscreen creams and lotions
 Daybreak 4329
 Apple Blossom 6564
 Muguet 4726
 Seloa Verde 6312
 Sandalwood 3708

Sunscreen oils
 Cassia PD0482
 Bouquet 6446 or 6637 or 6407

Perfumes for baby preparations

 Rose 4547
 Amaryllis 5103
 Lily of the Valley P2490

Perfumes for men's preparations

Pre-shave and after-shave lotions
 Valencia 6339
 Spice 6139
 Marquis 6352
 Sandalwood 3708

Brushless shaving cream
 Spruce Cologne 5497
 Hickory 5311
 Amberwood 6696
 Lemon Peel 6602

Information supplied by
NORDA SCHIMMEL

Perfumes for cosmetic lotions and creams

Bouquet French 2814
Hand Lotion Perfume
Floral Cream R249A
Chinese Bouquet
Rose for Cream A189
Violet K53059

Perfumes for shampoos

Almond Blossom R573A
Blue Hyacinth A311
Citrus Lime Bouquet A287
Lemon for Shampoo R540
Oriental Bouquet A253
Jasmin 55 for Cream Shampoo

Perfumes for deodorants

Fresh Lime for Men's Deodorant
Fougere
Floral Citrus Bouquet A211

Perfumes for men's cosmetics

Cedarwood R533
Lime and Leather A313
Sandal R6788
Spice Cologne A144
Tabac R19982
Woody Aroma 9547

COLOURS

BATH SALTS

D. F. Anstead (1 lb lots)

Water soluble Colours:
Pink 1658
Lemon Yellow 11104
Lavender 1677
Blue 1377

EYE COLOURS

(1) **D. F. Anstead** (1 lb lots)

Black 1430
Blue 1142
Green 11661
Brown 11928
Lavender 1677

(2) **Williams of Hounslow** (1 lb lots)

Cosmetic Green Oxide C61.6735
Cosmetic Blue C43.W1810
Cosmetic Mango, Violet C43.001
Cosmetic Black C33.134
Cosmetic Russet C3.128

LIPSTICK COLOURS

(1) **D. F. Anstead** (1 lb lots)

Eosin paste 25593
Rose paste 2535
Orange paste 25119

(2) **Williams of Hounslow** (1 lb lots)

Toning, Red, Dark C10.007
Sunburst Red C10.018
Dell Red C14.020   (other colours on demand)
Mystic Red Lake C14.023
Light Bromo C14.032
Manchu Orange C14.038

APPENDIX III

FACE POWDER COLOURS

Williams of Hounslow (1 lb lots)

Cosmetic tan C33.107
Cosmetic Sienna C33.123
Cosmetic Russett C33.128
Cosmetic Brown C33.115
Tangiers Orange C76.002
Persian Orange C74.003

(other colours for mixing and toning down can be obtained on application.)

EMULSION CREAMS, such as Foundation Creams

Similar colours to face powder colours.

Appendix IV
Addresses of suppliers

Alginate Industries
  Walter House, Bedford Street, London, W.C.2.

D. F. Anstead Limited
  Victoria House, Radford Way, Billericay, Essex.

Bio Cosmetic Limited
  High Street, Edgware, Middx.

The British Drug Houses
  Graham Street, City Road, London, N.1.

Bush, Boake, Allen Limited
  Ash Grove, London, E.8.

Rex Campell & Company
  7, Idol Lane, London, E.C.4.

Ciba Laboratories
  Horsham, Sussex.

Croda Limited
  24, Haymarket, London, S.W.1.

Evans Medical
  Bristol.

Glovers Chemicals Ltd
  Wortley Low Mills, Wortley. Leeds, 12.

Griffin Technical Studies
  P.O. Box 13, Wembley, Middlesex, HA0 1LD

Heyden Chemical Corporation
  8, Arthur Street, London, E.C.4.

Honeywell & Stein Limited
  (Atlas agent), Mill Lane. Carshalton, Surrey.

APPENDIX IV

Hopkinson & Williams
Freshwater Road, Chadwell Heath, Essex.

Imperial Chemical Industries Limited
Chemical Division, Local Regional Sales Office.

International Flavours & Fragrances
Crown Road, Southbury Road, Enfield, Middx.

Lankro Chemicals Limited
12, Whitehall, London, S.W.1.

Marchon Products Limited
Kells, Whitehaven, Cumberland.

Midland Silicones Limited
Reading, Berks.

Nipa Laboratories Limited
Treforest Trading Estate, Nr. Cardiff, Wales.

Norda-Schimmel International Limited
Stirling Road, Slough, Bucks.

Osborne Garrett & Company
Firth Street, London, W.1.

Proprietory Perfumes Limited
Ashford, Kent.

Pothe Hill & Company
Stratford, London, E.15.

Ronsheim & Moore
8, Buckingham Palace Gardens, London, W.C.1.

Samuelson & Company Limited
Roman Wall House, 1, Crutched Friars, London, E.C.3.

Shell Chemicals Company Limited
Shell House, London, S.W.1.

John & E. Sturge Limited
Wheeleys Road, Birmingham, 15.

Williams of Hounslow
Hounslow, Middx.

Appendix V
Glossary of scientific terms

AMINO-ACIDS. A group of organic compounds derived by replacing hydrogen atoms in the hydrocarbon (q.v.) groups of fatty acids (q.v.) or other organic acids with amino groups ($-NH_2$).

AMORPHOUS. Non-crystalline. Having no definite form or shape.

ANTIBODY. A protein produced in an animal when a certain kind of substance (ANTIGEN), which is normally foreign to its tissues, gains access to them. The formation of *antibodies* is a defence mechanism against invasion by bacteria and viruses.

ANTIOXIDANT. A chemical that prevents oxidation (q.v.) occuring.

AQUEOUS. Watery. Usually applied to solutions, indicating that the solvent is water.

AROMATIC COMPOUNDS. Organic compounds derived from benzene.

ELECTROLYTE. A compound which, in solution or the molten state, conducts an electric current and is, at the same time, decomposed by it. *Electrolytes* may be acids, bases or salts.

EMOLLIENT. An application that softens living tissue.

ESTERS. Organic compounds derived by replacing the hydroxylic hydrogen atom of an acid with a hydrocarbon (q.v.) group. For example $CH_3COOC_2H_5$ is the ethyl ester of acetic acid CH_3COOH.

FATTY ACIDS. Organic acids which have the general formula R.COOH, where R is a hydrogen atom or a hydrocarbon (q.v.) group.

HALOGENATED. Having an atom or atoms of one of the four elements, fluorine, chlorine, bromine or iodine, added to or substituted into the molecule.

HOMOGENEOUS. Of uniform composition throughout.

HOMOGENIZE. To make homogeneous (q.v.).

HYDROCARBON. A compound containing hydrogen and carbon only.

HYDROGENATED. Having been subjected to the chemical action of, or caused to combine with, hydrogen.

HYDROPHILIC. "Water loving". Certain groups of atoms in the molecules of organic compounds confer water solubility upon them. Such groups are said to be *hydrophilic*. The hydroxyl group (—OH) and the amino group (—NH_2) are common examples.

HYDROPHOBIC. "Water hating." The molecule of a detergent has not only a hydrophilic end-group but also a hydrocarbon chain which is soluble in fat and oil but insoluble in water. Such a chain is said to be *hydrophobic*.

LIPOPHILIC. "Oil loving". Part of the molecule soluble in oil.

LIPOPHOBIC. "Oil hating". Part of the molecule insoluble in oil.

OLFACTORY. Concerned with the sense of smell.

OXIDATION. Oxidation occurs when a substance combines with oxygen.

VISCOSITY. The property of a liquid whereby it tends to resist relative motion within itself. This is also shown by a tendency to resist the movement of solid objects in the liquid. Viscous liquids tend to be treacle-like.

Index of cosmetic formulae

Acne preparations (2)   *48*
After-shave lotions (4)   *63–4*
Anti-dandruff cream   *99*
Antiperspirants (6)   *71–2*
Astringent lotions (2)   *47–9*
Auburn hair rinse   *109*

Baby powders (3)   *77–8*
Barrier creams (2)   *50–1*
Bath oils (5)   *68–9*
Bath salts (2)   *66*
Bath salts, bubble   *66*
Bath, softening powder for the   *66*
Beauty masks   *90–2*
Black hair rinse   *110*
Brilliantines (3)   *106–7*

Casein mask   *90*
Cleansing and nourishing milk   *45*
Cleansing creams, emulsified (5)   *36–7*
                 liquifying (3)   *35*
Cleansing lotions (4)   *37*
Cold creams (12)   *32–4*
Cold creams (for removal of stage make-up) (3)   *121–2*
Cream bath   *67*
Cream mask for greasy skin   *92*
Cream mask, moisturizing   *92*
Cuticle creams (3)   *112*
Cuticle remover   *111*

Deodorants (5)   *69–70*
Dry skin cream   *44*
Dry skin lotion   *46*
Dusting powder, medicated   *78*

Eye liner   *80*
Eye shadows (4)   *78–80*
Eye shadow, powder   *80*

Face mask for dry skin   *91*
Face mask for greasy skin   *90*
Face powders (5)   *75, 77*
Foot bath salts (2)   *67*
Foot powders (2)   *78*
Foundation creams (9)   *41–3*
Fruit juice cream   *46*
Fuller's Earth mask   *91*

Gelatine mask *90*
Greasepaint,
    dry base for (3) *119*
    fat base for (3) *118–19*
    white *119–20*
    remover (2) *122*
Greasy skin, special creams for (3) *48–9*

Hair creams (18) *103–7*
Hair dyes (6) *108–10*
Hair setting lotions (2) *103*
Hand cleaning creams (6) *49–51*
Hand creams (8) *51–3*
Hand lotions (6) *53–5*
Henna hair dyes (2) *108*
Honey milk *45*

Lemon juice cream *46*
Lipsticks (10) *82, 85–8*
Liquid skin food *45*

Mascaras (4) *81–2*
Mask toners (2) *91*
Moisturizing creams (2) *44*
Milk bath *67*

Nail bleaches (2) *113*
Nail cream *112*
Nail varnish remover *113*
Nourishing milk *45*

Perfume, rose *16*

Rouges (7) *122–4*

Shampoos, cream (7) *96–9*
            jelly (3) *102–3*
            liquid (4) *100*
            lotion (4) *101*
Shaving creams, brushless (3) *60–1*
Shave lotions, pre-electric (3) *62–3*
Shaving soap cream *61*
Skin foods (2) *47*
Sunscreen cream base *56*
Sunscreen creams (2) *56–7*
Sunscreen/Insect repellent cream *58*
Sunscreen/Insect repellent lotion *58*
Sunscreen lotions (5) *57–8*
Sunscreen oil bases (2) *55–6*
Sun tan cream *59*
Sun tan oils (2) *59*

Talcum powders (8) 77–8
Tan and sunscreen cream 59
Toilet waters (3) 15
Toothpastes (5) 115–16
Tooth powders (2) 117
Vanishing creams (11) 39–41
Yeast mask 92

ADDITIONAL FORMULAE

ADDITIONAL FORMULAE

ADDITIONAL FORMULAE

ADDITIONAL FORMULAE